WILLIAM ACTON

PROSTITUTION

Edited, with an Introduction and Notes, by
PETER FRYER

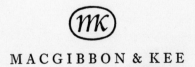

MACGIBBON & KEE

FIRST PUBLISHED LONDON 1857
FIRST PUBLISHED IN THIS EDITION 1968
BY MACGIBBON & KEE LIMITED
3 UPPER JAMES STREET GOLDEN SQUARE LONDON WI
COPYRIGHT © THIS EDITION MACGIBBON & KEE LTD 1968
PRINTED IN GREAT BRITAIN BY
COX & WYMAN LIMITED
LONDON, FAKENHAM AND READING

SBN: 261.62067.3

CONTENTS

CONTENTS

INTRODUCTION

THE DOMINANT attitude, a hundred years ago, to prostitution and the diseases it spread was pithily expressed by Samuel Solly (1805–71), Council member of the Royal College of Surgeons, Fellow of the Royal Society, and author of *The Human Brain* (1836). 'Far from considering syphilis an evil', he

> regarded it, on the contrary, as a blessing, and believed that it was inflicted by the Almighty to act as a restraint upon the indulgence of evil passions. Could the disease be exterminated, which he hoped it could not, fornication would ride rampant through the land. . . .

The best cure for syphilis, Solly added, was 'the elevation of the moral character of society'.*

In the eighteen-fifties, indeed, the subject of prostitution and the 'secret diseases' could hardly be mentioned outside the pages of the medical press. It so happens that we can pinpoint the year – the month, even – in which lay discussion began. In January 1858 the writer of a letter to the *British Medical Journal* on 'Public Prostitution' observed that 'but a few weeks ago . . . prostitution . . . did not admit of discussion; and yet today no less than two leading articles, and several letters, have appeared in the public journals'.† The writer was William Acton; and it was his own book on the subject, published in the previous year, which had done more than anything else to force the opening of a public debate on prostitution – and which was to challenge Solly's attitude in the name of one more rational, tolerant, and humane. By 1870, when the second edition of Acton's book appeared, though a speaker could tell the Social Science Congress that he 'preferred to see vice in the rags and filth of Whitechapel rather than in the silks and satins of the officer's mistress',‡ this kind of statement already had an old-fashioned and slightly irrelevant ring. To be sure, the Contagious Diseases Acts of 1864, 1866, and 1869, for which Acton had been one of the chief campaigners, and which provided for the medical examination of

---

* *Lancet*, 1860, I. 198. Solly was president of the Royal Medical and Chirurgical Society, 1867–68.
† *British Medical Journal*, 1858, 99.
‡ *Transactions of the National Association for the Promotion of Social Science, 1870* (1871), 227.

prostitutes in areas where there were naval and military stations,* were not only never extended to the civil population, as Acton urged, but were repealed eleven years after his death. Nevertheless Acton's iterated demand for the recognition, prevention, amelioration, and regulation of prostitution, and his awareness of its social causes – notably poverty and overcrowding – had a lasting and beneficial effect on public opinion.† Once started, the debate could not be suppressed; and it led before long to such a blow against hypocrisy as *Mrs Warren's Profession*, written in 1894 and first performed in the second year of the new century.

The book which opened the debate has not been reprinted since 1870, and its author sank, after his death five years later, into an obscurity from which Professor Steven Marcus has lately rescued him. Marcus describes Acton's *Prostitution* as 'a very good book, certainly the best piece of work of its kind from the period that I have read'.‡ The present edition makes this 'very good book' once more available to the general reader.

William John Acton was born in 1813 or, more probably, 1814 in Shillingstone (or Shilling Okeford), a quiet Dorset village in the valley of the Stour, about five miles north-west of Blandford Forum. Sources disagree about his date of birth. One says it was September 15, 1814;§ but this cannot be right, for the Shillingstone parish register shows he was baptized on May 12, 1814. The ceremony was performed by his father, Edward Acton, who had been curate of the parish since the previous October and was to bear that office for almost thirty years. In November 1817, when William was four, or almost four, his mother Elizabeth died, aged twenty-nine.

At seventeen, the boy went to London to study medicine, becoming an articled pupil of Charles Wheeler, apothecary to St Bartholomew's Hospital.‖ In 1836 he moved to Paris to continue his

---

* See note 1 on p. 232 below.

† See, e.g., Charles Booth's recommendation – in *Life and Labour of the People in London*, final vol. (1902), 128 – that houses of accommodation should be tolerated.

‡ Steven Marcus, *The Other Victorians* (New York, 1966), 4.

§ Frederic Boase, *Modern English Biography* (1892–1921), I. 12.

‖ Charles West Wheeler succeeded his father as apothecary to St Bartholomew's in 1821 and resigned in 1835.

education as *externe* – i.e. non-resident medical student acting as assistant or dresser – at the women's hospital for venereal diseases there, studying under the celebrated American-born venereologist Philippe Ricord (1800–89) and serving, in 1839, as secretary of the Parisian Medical Society. It was during Acton's pupilage that Ricord published his epoch-making *Traité pratique des maladies vénériennes* (Paris, 1838), in which gonorrhoea was clearly distinguished from syphilis for the first time and the characteristic phenomena of the three stages of syphilis were, for the first time, established.* To the end of his life, Acton considered Ricord his master, acknowledged his debt to him, and defended him from the attacks of medical men and others. Thus he protested energetically against the 'scandalous use' made of Ricord's name in quack advertisements proposing to restore the 'Vigour of Youth' in four weeks with 'Dr Ricord's Essence of Life', price 11s. (or 33s. for four quantities). 'The assumption of respectable names for the vilest purposes,' wrote Acton, 'is peculiar to Great Britain, and would not be submitted to in France.'†

As venereologists, Ricord and Acton were in advance of their immediate predecessors. But their methods were still to a great extent pre-scientific.‡ The gonococcus, the micro-organism that causes gonorrhoea, was not discovered till 1879; *Treponema pallidum* (or *Spirochaeta pallida*), the micro-organism that causes syphilis, not till 1905. The Wassermann test, the arsphenamines, bismuth

* An English translation, by H. P. Drummond, was published in 1842. Gonorrhoea had been separated from syphilis in 1793 by Benjamin Bell (1749–1806), but without Ricord's clarity and precision.

† *Lancet*, 1863, I. 527. 'Dr Ricord's Essence of Life' was sold by Prout & Co.'s Patent Medicine Warehouse, 229, Strand, London. It purported to cure impotence, nocturnal emissions, and nervous debility.

‡ There is no satisfactory general history of venereology. J. K. Proksch, *Die Geschichte der venerischen Krankheiten* (Bonn, 1895), is a biographical account (which includes, II. 765–6, a brief note on Acton). J. R. Whitwell, *Syphilis in Earlier Days* (1940), is concerned, like many other works, with theories of the origin of that disease, a reliable popular history of which will be found in James Cleugh, *Secret Enemy* (1954). W. A. Pusey, *The History and Epidemology of Syphilis* (Springfield, 1933), C. C. Dennie, *A History of Syphilis* (Springfield, [1962]), and Teodoro Pennacchia, *Storia della sifilide* (Pisa, 1961) are mere sketches, which may be supplemented by J. Johnston Abraham, 'Some Account of the History of the Treatment of Syphilis', *British Journal of Venereal Diseases*, XXIV

treatment, artificially induced malaria, and penicillin lay far in the future, as did the proof of the aetiological relationship of syphilis to general paralysis of the insane. Gonorrhoea was commonly treated by injecting a solution of silver nitrate into the urethra. For syphilis, mercury was a favourite treatment – one of Acton's earliest papers, read before the Parisian Medical Society, is entitled 'A Practical Essay on the Employment of Mercury in Syphilis'* – and was applied to the primary lesion in the form of oleate of mercury, or mercury with lanolin, and also swallowed in the form of grey powder, iodide of mercury, or corrosive sublimate. These doses tended to give patients a metallic taste in the mouth, sore gums, copious salivation, and bad breath; and the opponents of mercury treatment complained that it merely masked the symptoms, which tended to reappear in a modified form after the treatment was stopped. Acton made many contributions to the discussion, within the medical profession, on the practical aspects of his speciality. His first book, published a few months after his return to London in October 1840, was entitled *A Complete Practical Treatise on Venereal Diseases, and their Immediate and Remote Consequences* (1841).† It was the introductory chapter to the second (1851) edition of this work, separately printed as a 24-page pamphlet (*Prostitution in Relation to Public Health*, 1851), which formed the germ of his later book on prostitution.

Meanwhile Acton had become a Member of the Royal College of Surgeons (June 19, 1840); had begun practice in George Street, off Hanover Square, in 1840 (moving half a mile north to Queen Anne Street in November 1843); had been elected a Fellow of the Royal

---

* *Lancet*, 1839–40, I. 871–6.

† In the second (1851) and third (1860) editions the title was changed to: *A Practical Treatise on Diseases of the Urinary and Generative Organs (in Both Sexes)*.

(1948), 153–60. On the history of gonorrhoea, there are two short but useful surveys in *Annals of Medical History*: Edwin W. Hirsch, 'An Historical Survey of Gonorrhoea', n.s. II (1930), 414–23; and H. L. Wehrbein, 'Therapy in Gonorrhoea: an Historical Review', n.s. VII (1935), 492–7. An excellent conspectus of present-day diagnostic and therapeutic methods is Ambrose King, *Recent Advances in Venereology* (1964).

Medical and Chirurgical Society (1842); had been appointed surgeon to the Islington Dispensary (1845–46); and had begun to turn out a steady stream of medical papers, mostly for the *Lancet*. Even before the age of thirty, he was rapidly making a name for himself as writer and innovator. In November 1841 he exhibited to the Westminster Medical Society a new syringe for injecting silver nitrate into the urethra.* Syringes hitherto had been made of pewter or silver; Acton's, made entirely of glass, enabled the practitioner to see the amount of fluid he was about to inject. Moreover it had a glass bulb at the working end, instead of being pointed, and was accordingly less liable to injure the inflamed mucous membrane. Acton found his colleagues favoured far stronger solutions than he, often causing their patients intense pain and inflammation.† (Judging by Solly, some may have thought the pain edifying.)

'The Best Means of Disguising the Taste of Nauseous Medicines' was another subject to which Acton gave attention, along with smallpox in sheep, manufactured pasteboard splints, and the practice of withholding soldiers' pay while they were in hospital. In the eighteen-fifties, following a visit to Paris, he wrote several papers comparing venereological methods in the two capitals.

The year 1857 was his *annus mirabilis*. He addressed the inaugural Social Science Congress on prostitution (though his paper was printed last of all in the *Transactions*‡) and published two major books with characteristically sonorous titles: *The Functions and Disorders of the Reproductive Organs in Youth, in Adult Age, and in Advanced Life : Considered in their Physiological, Social, and Psychological Relations ;* and *Prostitution, Considered in its Moral, Social, & Sanitary Aspects, in London and Other Large Cities : with Proposals for the Mitigation and Prevention of its Attendant Evils.*§ Both books were well received, and the former was by far Acton's most successful production. A second edition came out in 1858, a third in 1862, and a sixth in the year of its author's death. *Functions and Disorders*

---

* A common specific for 'spermatorrhoea' (for which see note 36 on page 237 below) as well as gonorrhoea.

† Cf. *Lancet*, 1841–42, I. 272–3.

‡ *Transactions of the National Association for the Promotion of Social Science, 1857* (1858), 605–8.

§ Both titles were slightly changed in later editions. See the check-list of Acton's works, pp. 241–6 below.

is the book in which the best-known quotation from Acton is to be found, to the effect that most women, happily for them (or, as a later edition has it, happily for society) 'are not very much troubled with sexual feeling of any kind'.* The first edition has appendices on masturbation (which caused indigestion, loss of intellectual powers, pallor, emaciation, depression, and a taste for solitude, as well as 'the haggard expression, the sunken eye, the long, cadaver-ous-looking countenance, the downcast look') and on the copulative act in the bee; and 'hard-worked intellectual married men residing in London' are warned not to copulate more often than once a week, 'patients whose natural desires are strong' being advised 'to indulge in intercourse twice on the same night'.†

But however much Acton may have been the prisoner of the fictions of his age concerning female sexuality, masturbatory in-sanity,‡ and the need to avoid 'spending' one's semen too lavishly, his views on the social problems raised by the human sex drive in a prudish society were comparatively enlightened. He was the first, for instance, seriously to challenge the conventional parable that prostitutes necessarily rotted in ditches, died miserable deaths in workhouses, or perished in hospitals. Such a fate was exceptional, he insisted. Most prostitutes were transients, who re-entered the ranks of 'respectable' society within a very few years; and an increasing number did so by getting married, sometimes 'above their class'. Giving evidence before the House of Lords Select Committee on the Contagious Diseases Act in 1868, he was questioned on this point and took the opportunity of disabusing those of their Lord-ships who supposed that whores, when they 'lost [their] good looks' and retired, became brothel-keepers.§ As Marcus points out, 'all his recommendations for the treatment of prostitutes are in the direction of humanizing and rehabilitating them'.‖

And not only prostitutes, but women in danger of entering the

---

* Acton, *Functions and Disorders of the Reproductive Organs*, 3rd edition (1862), 101; 5th edition (1871), 115.

† *Ibid.* 1st edition (1857), 107–8, 56, 58, 108; 6th edition (1875), 188.

‡ Cf. E. H. Hare, 'Masturbatory Insanity: the History of an Idea', *Journal of Mental Science*, CVIII (1962), 1–25.

§ *Report from the Select Committee of the House of Lords on the Contagious Diseases Act, 1866* (1868), qq. 1059–60.

‖ Marcus, *op. cit.* 6.

profession. Expressing himself 'heart and soul' in favour of a scheme
for the redemption of 'fallen women' through employment as wet-
nurses, he answered critics in the following terms:

> Remember, it is not street-walkers nor professional prostitutes we
> are speaking of. We are speaking of the young house-maid or pretty
> parlour-maid in the same street in which the sickly lady has given birth
> to a sickly child, to whom healthy milk is life, and anything else death.
> With shame and horror the girl bears a child to the butler, or the police-
> man, or her master's son. Of course she is discharged; of course her
> seducer is somewhere else; of course, when her savings are spent, she
> will have to take, with shame and loathing, to a life of prostitution.
> Now, she is healthy and strong, and there is a little life six doors off,
> crying out for what she can give, and wasting away for the want of it,
> and in the nursing of that baby is a chance, humanly speaking, of her
> salvation from the pit of harlotry.

Such milk was not poison, and 'no accoucheur on the look-out for a
wet-nurse could be deceived into taking a syphilitic harlot'.*
Acton's speciality, and his appetite for public discussion of
hitherto forbidden topics, seem to have done his reputation no harm.
When his book on prostitution was first published, he was prepared
to have his proposals for reducing venereal diseases poohpoohed,
and to be roughly handled by the critics. On the whole, the critics
were kinder than he expected – except for one who complained that
'the style of the various chapters is very uneven, and in some respects
differs remarkably from that of Mr Acton's previous writing. Possibly this may be explained by an acknowledgment in the preface of
literary obligations to his *collaborateur*, Mr Horace Green'.† By
1868, Acton was pleased to find that 'most of the reforms I . . .

---

* 'Unmarried Wet-Nurses', *Lancet*, 1859, I. 175–6. Professor Marcus
(*op. cit.* 3) says he has 'not been able to obtain' this paper, but it could hardly
have been published less obscurely.

† *Medical Times and Gazette*, XXXVI (1857). 458. Cf. Acton, *Prostitution*, 1st edition (1857), p. ix, where Green is described also as 'my valued
friend, . . . whose energy and perfect appreciation of the objects I have in
view have been, I may truly say, invaluable to me'. Acton is possibly
referring to Horace Green (1802–66), first American physician to special-
ize in throat diseases, and author of several monographs. They could
have met during Green's second visit to Europe, in 1851.

advocated are about to be adopted'.* 'Mr Acton has never feared to touch pitch', wrote a medical reviewer of the third edition of *Functions and Disorders.*

> ... There are many men in the profession who would fear associating their name and reputation with discussions of this kind. But Mr Acton has undertaken to identify himself with all aspects of the sexual question, and it must be said that he has discussed them in this work with honesty, boldness, and manifest good intent.†

Only once, so far as I am aware, did Acton fall foul of his colleagues for making an indiscreet public statement. In 1868, addressing a mixed audience at the London Dialectical Society, he was reported as advising 'that ladies generally should use their influence with prostitutes to keep themselves clean, and to inspect the men with whom they had connexion'. Taken to task by the *British Medical Journal*, he explained rather weakly that he had thought the ladies present were midwives. 'What have midwives more than other women to do with prostitutes?' asked the *BMJ*.‡ Acton preferred not to reply.

He twice expressed strong views on subjects remote from his speciality. In the autumn of 1860, while staying in Brighton, he read a paper before the Medico-Chirurgical Society of that town 'On the Effects of Travelling on the Nervous System', and eighteen months later wrote to the *Lancet* on the same theme. He had observed that 'the stout, easy-going, lethargic traveller' could stand trains better than 'the spare, nervous, irritable man'. He himself, if he had to travel daily by rail, was obliged to restrict and regulate his diet. He could travel twenty miles a day each way on a well-laid line, doing this distance in forty minutes – 'but I would not venture so long a daily journey were the line notoriously bad, the carriage very shaky, or the speed excessive'. He had a practical suggestion for making travel more comfortable: that the transparent glass in railway-carriage windows be replaced with ground glass, to render objects outside invisible.§

---

* *British Medical Journal*, 1868, II. 153.
† *Lancet*, 1862, I. 518–19.
‡ *British Medical Journal*, 1868, II. 153.
§ *Lancet*, 1862, I. 210–11.

On his 1860 Brighton holiday, he had taken a house for eight weeks 'in one of those fine Eastern terraces facing the sea at Kemp Town'. The house-agent had told him the drainage was excellent. Within a fortnight however the drains stank, and the cook took to her bed for ten days with fever. One by one, his children and servants went down with headache, sickness, and 'febrile derangement'. His youngest child succumbed to a very severe form of diphtheria. The drainage of the house turned out to be 'wretchedly imperfect' – though the agent went on assuring him it was unobjectionable. Acton went to see the mayor, who confessed that Brighton had no public health officer; that the town's drainage was in a sorry state; and that for years he had been trying, without success, to get the town council to do something about it. Acton next complained to the Board of Health, who said they could do nothing unless an epidemic broke out. So he wrote a strong letter to the *Lancet*, taking 'the risk of damaging for the moment the pecuniary interests of the lodging-house keepers during this season, when the town is overflowing with fashionable society'. He added this mordant postscript: 'I regret to see in the obituary of *The Times*, the death of a distinguished officer from diphtheria, at a house in Brighton, only a short distance from my late residence.'*

The Times reprinted this letter,† and it caused a major sensation in Brighton. The town surveyor called Acton dishonest for basing a general charge on his domestic experiences; insisted there were excellent sewers and drains in Kemp Town; and questioned the connexion between diphtheria and bad drains. He did however admit that a large amount of sanitary work remained to be done in Brighton. Acton's house-agent weighed in with letters to *The Times* and the *Lancet*, repeating that the drains were perfectly satisfactory. To which Acton retorted: 'Within the last few days one of the "fine eastern terraces facing the sea" has furnished at least one little victim to what the Registrar-General has vigorously named "night-soil fever".'‡ And another *Lancet* correspondent, signing himself 'A Pure Air Seeker', came to Acton's support, telling how he had been driven out of Brighton by the stench of drains and cesspools,

* *Lancet*, 1860, II. 522.
† *The Times*, November 23, 1860, p. 10.
‡ *Lancet*, 1860, II. 571.

and describing his unavailing use of fumigations, eau-de-Cologne, and vinegar when the cesspool of the house next door was emptied:

> I was seized with sharp pains in the stomach, dizziness, nausea. . . . I left my landlady vomiting in her back parlour, *heard* her servant retching in the kitchen, and *saw* the old lady in the parlour attempting to sip brandy-and-water with a face like a poisoned cat.*

It was generally agreed that Acton had the better of the argument; but it was some time before Brighton's drains were improved.

Acton died in his bathroom at 17 Harley Street on December 7, 1875. For several weeks he had been unwell, and a post-mortem examination revealed the cause of death as fatty degeneration of the heart. His death provoked what was called 'an unnecessary display of energy'† on the part of Dr William Hardwicke, who had been coroner for central Middlesex for just over a year.‡ Acton's physicians held that an inquest was unnecessary, since the post-mortem findings corresponded with the symptoms exhibited during life and fully accounted for the mode of death. Their certificate did not sway the coroner, who insisted on an inquest. But a verdict of death from natural causes was returned.

Sir James Paget (1814–99), one of the greatest nineteenth-century surgeons and teachers, said of William Acton that he 'was careful and safe in practice, and had much technical skill'.

> Let it be remembered to his honour, that he practised honourably in the most dangerous of specialities; that he wrote decently on subjects not usually decent; and that he never used the opportunities which his practice offered for quackery or extortion. Even in those of his writings which related to social questions, and were, therefore, addressed in some measure to the public, there was nothing likely to serve his own interest; and he was always clearly on the side of morality.§

---

* *Lancet*, 1860, II. 571–2.

† *British Medical Journal*, 1875, II. 740.

‡ William Hardwicke (*c.* 1817–81), medical officer of health for Paddington and a pioneer of the idea of national insurance, wrote *On the Moral and Physical Advantages of Baths and Wash-Houses* (1874).

§ *Proceedings of the Royal Medical & Chirurgical Society*, VIII (1875–80), 75–6.

'Always clearly on the side of morality': this, it seems to me, is the secret of Acton's success – albeit a partial and in some ways temporary success – as a social reformer. He took care to remain well within the framework of the prevailing morality of his time and to utilize it, often skilfully, in support of his arguments. His *Prostitution* is as humane, as clear-sighted, above all as logical, as contemporary morality would permit.

In this, as in several other respects, it is much superior to any other nineteenth-century account of prostitution in this country. It is unnecessary to mention more than three. First, that ragbag of a book, *Prostitution in London* (1839) by Michael Ryan (1793–1840). Secondly, the section on 'La Prostitution en Angleterre' contributed by Gustave-Antoine Richelot (1807–93) to the 1857 edition of *De la prostitution dans la ville de Paris* by 'the Newton of Harlotry', A.-J.-B. Parent-Duchâtelet (1790–1836).* And thirdly, the more familiar section on 'Prostitution in London' contributed by 'Bracebridge Hemyng' (Samuel Bracebridge) to the 'extra volume' (*Those That Will Not Work*, 1862) of Henry Mayhew's *London Labour and the London Poor*. All three are derivative, exaggerated, and unworthy of the confidence social historians have placed in them. Ryan bases himself on the tendentious reports of various societies for the suppression of vice, which had a vested interest in exaggerating the number of prostitutes in London. Ryan's exaggerations were deplored, in his own day, by Dr Ralph Wardlaw,† the *Foreign Quarterly Review*, and the *London City Mission Magazine*.‡ Richelot

---

* It was Henry Milton who gave him this sobriquet, in an unsigned article in the *Quarterly Review*, LXX (1842), 20. I cannot refrain from quoting one further remark from Milton's review: 'To ascertain, within the fraction of an inch, the altitude, in an ascending series, of TWELVE THOUSAND FOUR HUNDRED AND FIFTY-FOUR Parisian prostitutes is a department of science, a species of philosophy, which we are convinced no human being but a Frenchman would ever have thought of cultivating' (*loc. cit.* 21 n.).

† In his *Lectures on Female Prostitution* (Glasgow, 1842), 141. Ralph Wardlaw (1779–1853) was professor of systematic theology at Glasgow University.

‡ 'Is it true that one out of every five females in London, between the ages of fifteen and fifty, including the highest, the middling, and the humbler classes, is a prostitute?' (*London City Mission Magazine*, IV (1839), 186 n.). The habit of wild exaggeration on this question went back to the metropolitan police magistrate Patrick Colquhoun. See note 12 on pp. 233–4 below.

relies on Ryan and on Léon Faucher's not conspicuously well-informed *Études sur l'Angleterre* (Paris, 1845). Mayhew's hack, in turn, simply plunders Ryan, Richelot – and Acton – and plumps for the ludicrous estimate of over 80,000 prostitutes in London. True, Acton himself is not above lifting an occasional fact or figure from Ryan, without acknowledgment; but the bulk of *Prostitution* is based on original study and observation. This makes Acton a great deal more accurate than Ryan and those who substantially rely on him.

Lastly, Acton is a more penetrating and powerful social observer than the others. 'One has to put up with the crude English method of development, of course', as Marx wrote of Darwin; but the detail is always convincing and often searing. *Prostitution*, so long neglected, is one of the basic documents of nineteenth-century English social history.

The present edition is abridged from the second, greatly expanded, edition of 1870. I have made three major cuts. In Chapter 3, 'Diseases the Result of Prostitution', much technical matter, of importance only to medical historians and other specialists, has been left out. From Chapter 5, which Acton calls 'Prostitution Abroad', I have retained only the material relating to France, and the chapter has been retitled accordingly. The detailed surveys of regulations in Belgium, Hamburg, Berlin, and Vienna, and of unregulated prostitution 'in the holy capital of sunny, passionate Italy', seemed to me to add little, if anything, to the argument. And Acton's Chapter 7, 'Recognition and Regulation of Prostitution in the Army and Navy', a subject dealt with more briefly elsewhere in the book, has been entirely omitted, later chapters being renumbered. Apart from that chapter, and sundry footnotes, all omissions are indicated by three full points (if short) or three asterisks (if long). In some places punctuation has been modernized. Editorial interpolations are enclosed in square brackets, as are several passages where word order has been changed for clarity's sake. Three of Acton's longer footnotes have been relegated to appendices, and a fourth appendix, giving the texts of two reviews (one of the first edition, the other of the second), has been added. Acton's footnotes, where retained, are indicated by conventional signs, as are a few additional references;

superior figures direct the reader to the editorial notes on pages 232–9. An elementary bibliographical apparatus has been provided, in the form of a list of the works quoted by Acton and a check-list of his own writings. The check-list is not, I fear, exhaustive; but all known editions and translations of his books and all his more important papers are included, as well as a fair selection of his letters to the leading medical journals.

It is a pleasure to acknowledge the help given me, in preparing this edition, by the staffs of the British Museum, the Dorset County Record Office, Dorchester, and the Wellcome Historical Medical Library, as well as by the Reverend William Eddleston, rector of Acton's native parish of Shillingstone.

P.F.

HIGHGATE, *9 March 1968*

AUTHOR'S PREFACE TO THE
SECOND EDITION

TWELVE years have elapsed since I submitted to public consideration the first edition of this work. I entered upon my labours with
feelings far different from those which induce me to resume them.
Then, the attempt to rouse attention to a question that seemed to
myself one of national importance, appeared almost hopeless. Now,
the mind and conscience of the nation are awakened, and opinions
which would have been formerly dismissed as idle dreams, are
deemed worthy of serious attention. During the intervening period
prostitution, with its attendant evils, has been the subject of anxious
inquiry. In 1864 the Secretary of State for War, and the Board of
Admiralty, appointed a Committee to report on the best means of
protecting the army and navy from the ravages occasioned by
venereal disease, and in 1866 an Act having this end in view – now
well known as the Contagious Diseases Act of 1866 – passed through
the legislature. The results achieved by means of this Act, and the
subject of prostitution generally, have also been reported on by two
Select Parliamentary Committees – one of the House of Lords, in
1868, the other of the House of Commons, in 1869 – and the legislature has seen fit to extend the scope of the Act of 1866, by an Act of
the last session.[1] . . . The working of this Act, and the public attention called to the subject, has been attended with the happiest
results, both as regards the health of our army and navy, and the
sanitary and moral improvement wrought in the unhappy women
who have come within the scope of its provisions. So much so, that
we read in the report of the above-mentioned Committee of the
House of Commons:

> Although the Act has only been in operation two years and a half,
> and at some stations only seven months, strong testimony is borne to
> the benefits, both in a moral and sanitary point of view, which have
> already resulted from it.
>
> Prostitution appears to have diminished, its worst features to have
> been softened, and its physical evils abated.*

* [*Report from the Select Committee on Contagious Diseases Act (1866)*
(1869), p. iii.]

This Act, however, is something more than a means of imparting health both physical and moral. It forms the commencement of a new legislative era, being a departure from that neutral position previously held by English law with respect to venereal diseases, and admits that there is nothing in the nature of prostitution to exclude it from legislative action, but that, on the contrary, it may be necessary to recognize its existence, and to provide for its regulation, and for the repression, so far as possible, of its attendant evils. It is, in fact, the adoption – so far as it goes – of the principle for which I have always contended, that prostitution ought to be an object of legislation.

I believe I may claim, without vanity, to have in some measure paved the way for, and guided the progress of, this change, and I hail with satisfaction the advent of the time which has at length arrived when we may contemplate work accomplished, and, guided by the experience gained from results attained, consider what more remains to be achieved.

Although the benefits that have resulted from the recent legislation – as regards this special class of disease – are undoubted, there is great unwillingness in certain quarters to extend them from a class to the nation, and a radical distinction is sought to be drawn between the case of the army and navy and that of the civil population. Strange as it may appear, the same arguments that were urged against interference by the legislature with venereal maladies previously to the passing of the Contagious Diseases Bill – of whose futility that measure is the strongest possible acknowledgment – are still put forward with as much confidence as though they had never received such authoritative refutation, and must still be met and answered, so fas as the civil population is concerned. Opposition to legislative interference is still based mainly on religious and moral grounds, the risk of encouraging sin, and the injustice of curtailing individual freedom. I yield to no man in my love of liberty and regard for religion. I am therefore especially careful in the following pages to show that the interference which I propose with personal liberty is unhappily necessary both for the sake of the community at large, and of the women themselves. Such interference is, in fact, not special – it is the extension to venereal disorders of the principle on which the Government endeavours to act in dealing with other forms of preventable disease. Nor have the objections on religious grounds to the course which I propose any real foundation; on the contrary, religion is on my side.

The fresh phase assumed by the question discussed in the ensuing pages has necessitated considerable changes and modifications on my part, and I find that much of the matter contained in my first edition may now be conveniently omitted. The whole work has been carefully revised and remodelled, and to a great extent rewritten; moreover, sources of information formerly closed or unknown, are now open to me. My statistics are no longer solely dependent on my own opportunities for investigation. I have been enabled to make use of the researches of others, and much official assistance has been accorded to me. I have described the actual state of prostitution at home and abroad, and have shown the different methods of dealing with it employed in this and other countries, thus rendering easy the comparison between the state of things existing in England and on the Continent, and the rival systems of legislation prevailing here and there.

It will be seen that on a great part of the Continent the necessity for the RECOGNITION of prostitution by the State, and the adoption of remedial and preventive measures, has long been acknowledged, while in England such recognition has been, till within the last few years, steadily refused, and is now conceded only in the exceptional case of the army and navy. The Continental system, owing to the way in which police supervision is there carried out, has been termed the licensing system; the English, under which prostitutes [are left to themselves (except in districts to which the Contagious Diseases Act applies)] has been termed the voluntary system.

In considering the attitude which it becomes us to assume towards prostitution, one fact must be carefully borne in mind: that it is no evanescent evil, but that it has existed from the first ages of the world's history down to the present time, and differs but little, and in minor particulars, in this the nineteenth century, from what it was in the earliest times. The records of the human race, from the Book of Genesis downwards, through the whole range of ancient and medieval literature to the writings of our own day, bear witness to the perpetual presence among men of the daughters of shame. Kings, philosophers, and priests, the learned and the noble, no less than the ignorant and simple, have drunk without stint in every age and every clime of Circe's cup; nor is it reasonable to suppose that in the years to come the world will prove more virtuous than it has shown itself in ages past. From time to time men's purer instincts, revolting from the sin, have striven to repress it; but such efforts have too often ended in failure, and entailed disasters more terrible than those from which relief was sought; and it is evident that it would be unreasonable to expect any other result. Equally irrational is it to imagine that this irrepressible evil can exist without entailing upon society serious mischief; though incapable of absolute repression, prostitution admits of mitigation. To ignore an ever-present evil appears a mistake as fatal as the attempt to repress it. I am, therefore, an advocate of RECOGNITION.

It is high time for us to get the better of 'a fear that starts at shadows'. This word RECOGNITION may sound very dreadful, and be regarded by many as the precursor of a coming deluge of continental immorality. But what is the real fact? Is not recognition already accorded by society? Who are those fair creatures, neither chaperons nor chaperoned, 'those somebodies whom nobody knows', who elbow our wives and daughters in the parks and promenades and rendezvous of fashion? Who are those painted, dressy women, flaunting along the streets and boldly accosting the passers-by? Who those miserable creatures, ill-fed, ill-clothed, uncared for, from whose misery the eye recoils, cowering under dark arches and among bye-lanes? The picture has many sides; with all of them society is more or less acquainted. Why is the State – that alone can remedy a condition of things that all deplore – alone to refuse recognition? The voluntary system has been tried long enough with its affected ignorance and empty parade of hospitals, penitentiaries, and asylums. Individual efforts are powerless to effect either the cure of disease or the reformation of the prostitute. The nation's weakness can be assisted only by the nation's strength; and I propose to show that concentrated effort, sanctioned by authority, can alone stay the ravages of a contagious and deadly disorder, and that only by methodical and combined action, and by gradual and almost imperceptible stages, can any moral cure be effected.

To the licensing system of the Continent I am as strongly opposed for the reasons given in the text as I am to the voluntary system hitherto adopted in England – the necessary consequence of the neutral position assumed by the legislature. My examination of the character of prostitution – the causes that produce [it] and the evils that result from it – leads me to this conclusion: that the consequences of RECOGNITION must be threefold, and embrace PREVENTION, AMELIORATION, and REGULATION. For the sake of greater clearness I have devoted a separate chapter to each of these three divisions.

Although some of the causes of prostitution are undoubtedly beyond the reach of legislation, others are clearly amenable to it. To these last I address myself in the chapter on Prevention. Thus I propose to diminish the amount of prostitution by putting an end so far as possible to the overcrowding of families, and making better provision for the relief and suitable employment of women. With this object also I propose to remodel the laws relating to seduction, making the seducer substantially responsible for the support of his bastard offspring – providing facilities for procuring affiliation orders – and assisting the pregnant woman during her confinement. Such legislation would, I am fully persuaded, diminish the number of seductions by increasing the responsibility thereto attaching, and would as a necessary consequence decrease the amount, not only of prostitution but also of ILLEGITIMACY and INFANTICIDE. With this object, I demand that the funds of the Foundling Hospital, producing as they now do an annual revenue of the present value of £11,000, and an assured income within the present century (according to the Charity Commissioners) of £40,000 a year, shall for the future be applied more in accordance with the intention of the founder than they are at present.[2]

I could hardly have avoided, had I wished to do so, alluding to the kindred subjects of ILLEGITIMACY, BABY-FARMING, and INFANTICIDE, following as they do, with prostitution, in the wake of seduction. It seems to me that all these forms of evil, germane to and dependent on each other, should be the subjects of legislation, and I have gladly availed myself of the opportunity of pointing out the direction which that legislation should in my opinion take. It seems to me that the mischiefs attendant on SEDUCTION, PROSTITUTION, and ILLEGITIMACY, require careful and comprehensive handling. These evils are all to a certain extent preventable, and the agency to which any one of them is amenable is capable of dealing with all the rest. I propose the formation of a GOVERNMENT BOARD, to which might be intrusted the working of the amended bastardy laws and the Contagious Diseases Act, the care of illegitimate children, and the amelioration of fallen women. By this means the various evil consequences of seduction would be subjected to that methodical and organized action which it seems to me essential to provide, if we desire to deal effectually with evils too vast and too difficult for private enterprise. To the preventive measures advocated in the following pages I apprehend little hostility, as it is agreed on all hands that the temptations to adopting a life of prostitution should be removed as far as possible; but when I insist upon the duty of REGULATION and AMELIORATION, I find that my more timid friends fall away from me, and accuse me of countenancing sin, and of encouraging people in immorality by making the consequences of their evil ways less painful and degrading. I repudiate this unjust accusation as a cruel calumny, and am sure that no impartial reader, after examining my proposals, and the reasons by which I support them, will consider it to be well founded. It seems to me vain to shut our eyes to the fact that prostitution must always exist. Regret it as we may, we cannot but admit that a woman if so disposed may make profit of her own person, and that the State has no right to prevent her. It has a right, however, in my opinion, to insist that she shall not, in trafficking with her person, become a medium of communicating disease, and that, as she has given herself up to an occupation dangerous to herself and others, she must, in her own interest and that of the community, submit to supervision. My proposals go to this extent, and no further – viz., to make the evil that we cannot repress as little injurious as possible. I desire to protect both society at large, and the individual, from the permanent injury at present inflicted by a highly contagious and virulent disorder. I desire also to heal the sick prostitute, and to cleanse her moral nature. The State must moreover set its face against anyone, man or woman, making a profit of another's prostitution. I may here observe that it unhappily appears necessary to extend toleration to persons who keep accommodation-houses; otherwise hotels, coffee-houses, and other places of public resort will become debased.

If, in spite of all the precaution that can be taken, the woman becomes a prostitute, our next object should be to attempt to ameliorate her condition, so as to enable her to pass through this stage of her existence with as little permanent injury to herself and as little mischief to society as possible. This is the more important because I prove that the great mass of prostitutes in this country are in course of time absorbed into the so-called respectable classes, and

I maintain that in proportion as they are assisted or neglected during their evil days will they assume the characters of wives and mothers with a greater or less degree of unsoundness in their bodies and pollution in their minds. Notwithstanding the incalculable importance of working such reformation as may be possible in these unhappy women, no adequate effort in this direction has ever yet been made, and it is a lamentable fact that while the penitentiaries and asylums on the one hand effect but little good, and are at once expensive and useless, on the other the present hospital system is inadequate to the task of coping with the diseases incidental to prostitution.

To give access to and control over the woman whose amelioration we desire to accomplish, it seems to me absolutely necessary that the Contagious Diseases Act should be extended to the civil population, for by means of its machinery alone can we discover and detain till cured the women afflicted with syphilitic diseases, and in no other way that has occurred to me can the supervision necessary for enabling us to work a gradual improvement in their lives be obtained. In our efforts to ameliorate the prostitute, we must doubtless tolerate much that we would willingly discountenance, but of two evils we must choose the least.

In the consideration as to the advisability of extending the above-mentioned Act, the expenditure that must be thereby incurred, though not a primary [element], is undoubtedly an important [one]. I have entered fully into the necessary calculations, and I believe that the figures which I have placed before my readers will convince them that the expenditure will be moderate, when weighed with the benefits obtained.

The reader who is a conscientious parent must perforce support me; for, were the sanitary measures I advocate once in operation, with what diminished anxiety would he not contemplate the progress of his boys from infancy to manhood? The statesman and the political economist are mine already, for are not armies and navies invalidated – is not labour enfeebled – is not even population deteriorated by the evils against which I propose we should contend? The sympathies of all who can look kindly upon the sick, the sorry, and the fallen, must gain new impulse from the study of the facts, figures, and deductions, possibly new to them, which I have here marshalled for their use.

I shall have occasion, in the body of the text, to express my thanks to several gentlemen whose communications I have turned to good account. My public acknowledgment is more especially due to Lord Stanley,[3] who – with the ready appreciation of a true statesman – at once saw the importance of the Continental information I sought for, and willingly instructed our ministers at the different foreign Courts to collect . . . statistics. . . .

To the Registrar General, and to my kind friend, Dr Farr,[4] I beg to tender my thanks for the correction of tables, which, without their assistance, I could not have obtained. To Captain Harris,[5] Assistant Commissioner of Police, I here acknowledge my indebtedness, and to many others to whom I have submitted my proof-sheets, and who, in authenticating the correctness of their statements, have added so much to the value of this book.

17 QUEEN ANNE STREET,
November 1869

I

PROSTITUTION DEFINED

ETYMOLOGY would, of course, at once suggest a 'standing forth, or plying for hire in open market', as a definition of the word prostitution. Charitable and refined persons instinctively recoil from its general use, under the very natural impression that the essence of 'prostitution' is not so much *the receipt of consideration* as *community*; but, on the other hand, many forcible divines and moralists have maintained that all illicit intercourse is prostitution, and that this word is as justly applicable as those of 'fornication' and 'whoredom' to the female who, whether for hire or not, voluntarily surrenders her virtue. According to them, her first offence is as much an act of prostitution as its repetition.

For the purpose of the politico-statistical researches which the French administrators have, since the time of the first Republic, made into prostitution, as well as everything else, they arrange disorderly women under two heads, *femmes débauchées* and *prostituées*. The former, instead of being, as would at first sight appear, a generic term, seems to distinguish the numerous group known as *femmes galantes* and *filles clandestines*, and corresponds with the 'kept mistresses' and more reserved class of prostitutes in this country. Over it, while a certain degree of self-respect is preserved, the police neither assert nor can maintain control. Its members enjoy to the full extent their civic rights, and a maxim of law is acknowledged in their favour, which their sisters of this country are obliged to maintain for themselves – often to the disgust, and occasionally to the amusement, of the public. . . .

Into the second class, which answers to our common street-walkers, the French authorities do their best to drive such of the first as they consider to have forfeited their independent position. It is held that the legally established and repeated exercise of fornication as a calling, combined with public notoriety thereof, arrest *in flagrante*, proved by witnesses other than the informer or the police agent, constitute the 'prostitute'. . . .

PROSTITUTION

According to the Board of Public Morals at Berlin, all voluntary sexual abandonment for a consideration is held to be prostitution. The necessity of defining not only 'a prostitute' but 'a common prostitute' may be seen from a perusal of the evidence on which is formed the report of the Select Committee on the Contagious Diseases Act, . . . published . . . July 1869 . . .

> *The Chairman, the Hon. J. C. Vivian*:[6] What other new clause would you propose? – *Mr Sloggett,*[7] *Visiting Surgeon to the Devonport Lock Hospital* . . .: I think that a new clause should be introduced defining more exactly the term 'common prostitute'.
>
> What clause is there in this Bill which defines the term 'common prostitute'? – There is no such clause.
>
> How would you propose to define a common prostitute? – I would first define them as women who habitually gain their livelihoods, partly or wholly, by the proceeds of prostitution.
>
> *Sir John Pakington*:[8] Is there in the law of England no definition of a prostitute? – I think not. . . .
>
> *Dr Brewer*:[9] What is your definition of a prostitute? . . . *Mr Parsons,*[10] *Visiting Surgeon to the Portsmouth Lock Hospital* . . .: Any woman whom there is fair and reasonable ground to believe is, first of all, going to places which are the resorts of prostitutes alone and at times when immoral persons only are usually out. It is more a question as to mannerism than anything else.
>
> Must she be making her livelihood by it? – Yes, she ought to be; but, if you confine yourself to that definition, all I can tell you is, that your Act will never succeed. The amount of clandestine prostitution is very large. I think the definition here, of 'common prostitute', is very objectionable, inasmuch as I have heard it stated, by those who wish to object to the Act, that you have no right to bring under the provisions of the Act what may be called the better class of prostitutes, who, they say, are not common prostitutes.*

Mr John Simon,[11] the Medical Officer . . . to the Privy Council, said, in reply to a question . . . put to him:

> . . . How are you to prove clandestine prostitution? Would those who propose such things take a woman on the mere ground of her having

* [*Report from the Select Committee on Contagious Diseases Act* (*1866*) (1869), qq. 158–61, 374–75.]

had sexual relations with more than one man, and put two and two together, and produce their evidence in a police court? It seems to me to be a thing which could not be done; the only kind of prostitution which can be dealt with, I suppose, is prostitution carried on by women who make it their calling, and live in gangs in brothels, or who publicly solicit men. I do not see any practical definition of prostitution which could include women wishing to practise clandestinely.*

Leaving those on whom the duty of passing acts of Parliament devolves to discover the definition necessary for their purpose, I shall here content myself with a definition sufficiently accurate to point out the class of persons who ought, in my opinion, to become the objects of legislation, and shall assume, for the purpose of my present inquiry, that the fact of 'hiring', whether openly or secretly, whether by an individual or a plurality in succession, constitutes prostitution.

* [*Ibid.* q. 1301.]

2

PROSTITUTION IN ENGLAND

To obviate the possibility of misapprehension, I remind the reader that I regard prostitution as an inevitable attendant upon civilized, and especially closely-packed, population. When all is said and done, it is, and I believe ever will be, ineradicable. Whether its ravages, like those of disease and crime, may not be modified by unceasing watchfulness – whether it may not be the duty of the executive, as a French writer suggests, to treat it as they do such ordinary nuisances as drains, sewers, and so forth, by diminishing its inconvenience to the senses, and, in fact, rendering its presence as little noticeable as possible – it will be my business to inquire in a future chapter. In the present I shall offer as complete a survey of that portion of it which stalks abroad, *tête levée* [with head erect], in this metropolis, and other parts of the kingdom, as the facts at any English writer's disposal admit of.

The number of prostitutes in London has been variously estimated, according to the opportunities, credulity, or religious fervour of observers, and the width of interpretation they have put upon the word. To attempt to reconcile or construct tables upon the estimates I have met with would be a hopeless task. I can merely give a few of the more moderate that have been handed down by my predecessors. Mr Colquhoun,[12] a magistrate at the Thames Police Court, rated them at 50,000 some sixty years ago. The Bishop of Exeter[13] spoke of them as reaching 80,000; Mr Talbot,[14] secretary of a society for the protection of young females, made the same estimate. The returns on the constabulary force presented to Parliament in 1839, furnished an estimate of 6,371 – viz., 3,732 'known to the police as kept by the proprietors of brothels', and 2,639 as resident in lodgings of their own, and dependent on prostitution alone for a livelihood. It was estimated by the Home authorities in 1841, that the corresponding total was 9,409 – which, I need hardly point out, does not include the vast numbers who regularly or occasionally abandon themselves, but in a less open manner.

I am indebted to the courtesy of Sir Richard Mayne,[15] the late Chief Commissioner of Metropolitan Police, for the subjoined return, as well as for those of 1837 (made up in 1841):

A Return of the number of Brothels and Prostitutes within the Metropolitan Police District, as nearly as could be ascertained at that date (May 20th, 1857).

Division	Number of Brothels					Number of Prostitutes			
	Where prostitutes are kept	Where prostitutes lodge	Where prostitutes resort	Total	Total returned in 1841	Well dressed, living in brothels	Well dressed, walking the streets	Low, infesting low neighbourhoods	Total
A	—	—	—	—	—	—	—	—	—
B	—	135	18	153	181	16	144	364	524
C	14	92	46	152	83	168	150	—	318
D	10	113	16	139	93	49	188	289	526
E	30	110	54	194	266	74	85	387	546
F	26	—	19	45	181	60	120	300	480
G	3	77	27	152	360	26	165	158	349
H	209	217	45	471	289	132	420	1251	1803
K	—	402	17	419	882	13	435	517	965
L	—	184	193	377	275	108	329	365	802
M	12	138	28	178	178	13	71	583	667
N	53	98	34	185	152	87	142	216	445
P	3	33	29	65	56	63	67	98	228
R	46	66	36	148	122	69	116	216	401
S	—	52	36	88	96	8	90	133	231
T	—	12	—	12	107	—	12	94	106
V	4	37	6	47	4	35	82	92	209
Total	410	1766	649	2825	3325	921	2616	5063	8600
Do. 1841	933	1544	848	3325	—	2071	1994	5344	9409

A. Whitehall, the Parks, Palaces, Government Offices.
B. Westminster, Brompton, Pimlico, part of Chelsea.
C. St James's, Regent-street, Soho, Leicester-square.
D. Marylebone, Paddington, St John's Wood.
E. Between Oxford-street, Portland-place, New-road, and Gray's-inn-lane.
F. Covent Garden, Drury-lane, St Giles's.
G. Clerkenwell, Pentonville, City-road, Shoreditch.
H. Spitalfields, Houndsditch, Whitechapel, Ratcliff.
K. Bethnal-green, Mile-end, and from Shadwell to Blackwall.

L. Lambeth and Blackfriars, including Waterloo-road, &c.
M. Southwark, Bermondsey, Rotherhithe.
N. Islington, Hackney, Homerton, &c.
P. Camberwell, Walworth, part of Peckham.
R. Deptford, Greenwich, and neighbourhood.
S. Kilburn, Portland, Kentish and Camden Towns to Cattle Market.
T. Kensington, Hammersmith, North End, Fulham.
V. Walham-green, Fulham, Chelsea, Cremorne.

The headings of the above table demand a few explanatory observations. It is, in the first place, desirable that the reader should understand the distinction between the three classes of houses, termed by the police, brothels. The first, or 'houses in which prostitutes are kept', are those whose proprietors overtly devote their establishments to the lodging, and sometimes to the boarding, of prostitutes, and prostitutes only. At first sight it might appear that, by the phrase employed, were indicated houses in which prostitutes are harboured, fed, and clothed at the cost of speculators, who derive a revenue from the farm of their persons. Such is, however, not the intention of the framers of the document. The houses last mentioned are, doubtless, included in the first column of the above returns, but [as will be seen in the next table] these have now almost disappeared from the Metropolis.

By 'houses in which prostitutes lodge', the reader must understand those in which one or two prostitutes occupy private apartments, generally with, though perhaps in rare cases without, the connivance of the proprietor. It often occurs, it must be remembered, that females of no virtue are so desirous of preserving the appearance of it before those among whom they reside that they will not introduce their paramours to their apartments; but both they and their domicile, being generally known to the police, both figure on the return. 'Houses to which prostitutes resort' represent night houses – the brothels devoted to casual entertainment of these women and their companions, and the coffee-shops and supper-shops which they haunt.

The 'well-dressed, living in lodgings' prostitute is supposed to be the female who, though to all intents and purposes common, extending her pursuit of acquaintances over the town at large, or limiting it to the places of public recreation, eschews absolute 'street-walking'.

The 'well-dressed, walking the streets' is the prostitute errant, or absolute street-walker, who plies in the open thoroughfare and there only, restricting herself generally to a definite parade, whereon she may always be found by her friends, and hence becomes, of course, 'perfectly well known to the police'.

The 'low prostitute, infesting low neighbourhoods', is a phrase which speaks for itself. The police have not attempted to include – in fact, could not have justly included, I might almost say – the unnumbered prostitutes whose appearance in the streets as such never takes place; who are not seen abroad at unseemly hours; who are reserved in manners, quiet and unobtrusive in their houses or lodgings, and whose general conduct is such that the most vigilant of constables could have no pretence for claiming to be officially aware of their existence or pursuits. The 1869 Report on the Contagious Diseases Act enables us for the first time to show the proportions of common prostitutes to soldiers at Aldershot. Thus, Inspector Smith[16] gave in a report proving that there were in June 1869, 243 recognized prostitutes to about 12,000 troops. This paucity of prostitutes, according to Dr Barr,[17] causes some of them to have intercourse with 20 or 23 men in one night.*

The falling off (amounting almost to extinction of the class) of the number of 'houses where prostitutes are kept', which is shown by the table of 1868, cannot fail to strike the reader, the number given being two only as against 410 in 1857 and 933 in 1841. It appears that of the eleven prostitutes returned, as inhabiting such houses, one only resides in one of these houses, and ten in the other; this latter is kept by a Frenchwoman. It is satisfactory to find that this class of house is, if we may trust the police, rapidly disappearing from London. It is not too much to say that the brothel where prostitutes are kept is an institution alien to English feelings, and that even if the government should sanction the maintenance of such houses, which is far from probable, public opinion may be confidently expected to work their extinction. I may here call attention to a lesson taught us pretty clearly by these returns, which is, that to attempt to put down prostitution by law is to attempt the impossible. Notwithstanding the numerous prosecutions and parish raids which have been directed against prostitutes and their dwellings during the past few

---

* [*Report from the Select Committee on Contagious Diseases Act (1866)* (1869), q. 751.]

years, there were in the year 1868, 1,756 houses where prostitutes lodge, against 1,766 in 1857. What can show more strongly the impossibility of [suppressing prostitution by the arm of the law]? Eleven years ago I pointed out that if a prostitute is prosecuted for plying her trade in one parish, she will only move into another. The result has proved the truth of my prediction, and recent failures add their testimony to that of world-wide experience, and prove the impolicy of making attempts of this nature, except in cases when the houses proceeded against are shown to be productive of open scandal or a cause of intolerable annoyance.

I must observe that these returns give but a faint idea of the grand total of prostitution by which we are oppressed, as the police include in them only those women and houses whose nature is well and accurately known to them. There can be little doubt that numbers of women who live by prostitution lead apparently respectable lives in the lodgings or houses which they occupy; but all such are necessarily excluded from the returns.

Were there any possibility of reckoning all those in London who would come within the definition of prostitutes, I am inclined to think that the estimates of the boldest who have preceded me would be thrown into the shade.

* * *

Having briefly called attention to the vast extent of the evil with which we have to contend, I will now endeavour to supply the reader with some general idea of the unfettered domestic life and haunts of London prostitutes, which, in default of better experience, we can presently bring to bear, with what information we may have as to the present state of our law, towards estimating the practicability of assimilating it to any of the laws which prevail abroad, or otherwise improving it. For the sake of clearness, I shall briefly notice under separate heads:

1. HOMES – viz., *dress houses; houses in which prostitutes lodge.*

2. HAUNTS – viz., *introducing houses; accommodation houses; casinos and pleasure gardens; the public streets.*

Dress Houses. – The description of brothels called dress houses was much more prevalent a few years ago than is the case at present. It appears from the police returns for 1868, that there are now only two such houses in the Metropolis, containing between them 11 inmates.* They were maintained to some extent by persons who furnished board, lodging, and clothes to a number of prostitutes whom they sent out into the streets under guard of servants, or kept at home to receive visitors. The girls, who, it is needless to say, were of the most utterly degraded class, received but a small share of the wages of their sin; their condition was almost as abject as the *filles numérotées* of the Continent in general, and they were far more unprotected than those of Berlin, especially against persons speculating in them. The spread of venereal taint was not, as might be imagined, more favoured by this most revolting phase of the evil than by any other. The brutalized woman-farmers had, it is true, no more bowels of compassion for the male sex than for their stock-in-trade, and would drive into the streets with taunts and curses the diseased unfortunate. But the evil reputation which an establishment might acquire by being a focus of disease, induced them to adopt a certain degree of care and precaution. To show, however, the dangers to which the unwary might be exposed under that system, I may mention a case that came under the notice of a friend of my own.

In the year 1858 his sympathy and curiosity were awakened by the behaviour of a very handsome girl, who, seemingly against her will, was very urgently forced upon his notice by a brothel-keeper, who was hawking her about the streets. Acquiescing in the offer of her company and paying the demands of the house, he put some searching questions to the girl. She at first half confessed slight indisposition, but on his avowing himself a medical man, and showing clearly enough that his curiosity like his gift was dictated by mere charity, she submitted to a superficial examination. No more was required to prove that she was a mass of syphilis.

The rouged and whitewashed creatures, with painted lips and eyebrows, and false hair, accustomed to haunt Langham Place, portions of the New Road, the Quadrant, the Peristyle of the Haymarket Theatre, the City Road, and the purlieus of the Lyceum, were the most prominent gangs of this description in London. They were watched by persons of their own sex, employed purposely to prevent their abstraction of the lodging-house finery, and clandestine traffic

---

* I am informed that the exception in London is the rule in Edinburgh. It will appear in a subsequent chapter, there is less disease in brothels conducted on the French principle than among isolated prostitutes. I do not know whether the Scotch brothels can boast a similar advantage.

RETURN OF THE NUMBER OF BROTHELS AND PROSTITUTES IN EACH
METROPOLITAN POLICE DIVISION, 1868

Police Division	Number of Brothels and Places					Number of Prostitutes			
	Where Prostitutes are kept	Where Prostitutes lodge	Where Prostitutes resort	Coffee Houses or other Places where Business is ostensibly carried on, but which are known to the Police to be used as Brothels or places of accommodation for Prostitutes	Total	Well-dressed living in Brothels	Well-dressed living in Private Lodgings	In low Neighbourhoods	Total
A. or Whitehall	—	—	—	—	—	—	—	—	—
B. Westminster	—	141	2	18	161	—	167	310	477
C. St James's	—	106	1	21	128	—	227	10	237
D. Marylebone	—	7	3	15	25	—	128	162	290
E. Holborn	1	171	8	11	191	10	371	136	517
F. Covent Garden	1	—	1	21	23	1	2	427	430
G. Finsbury	—	86	35	13	134	—	29	235	264
H. Whitechapel	—	126	2	11	139	—	—	623	623
K. Stepney	—	350	9	16	375	—	133	799	932
L. Lambeth	—	149	34	21	204	—	144	228	372
M. Southwark	—	19	23	19	61	—	14	314	328
N. Islington	—	127	—	15	142	—	247	186	433
P. Camberwell	—	43	1	4	48	—	—	65	65
R. Greenwich	—	125	6	12	143	—	144	415	559
S. Hampstead	—	—	—	5	5	—	128	45	173
T. Kensington	—	193	1	4	198	—	236	110	346
V. Wandsworth	—	12	—	—	12	—	33	85	118
W. Clapham	—	27	—	1	28	—	23	53	76
X. Paddington	—	23	1	6	30	—	61	50	111
Y. Highgate	—	51	5	16	72	—	68	96	164
Total	2	1756	132	229	2119	11	2155	4349	6515

with men. These wretched women, virtually slaves, though nominally free, with bodies and time no longer their own, were restricted, for the convenience of the real proprietors, to certain parades or beats, and from year's end to year's end might be observed on the same side of one particular street, and within a few hundred yards or less of one particular spot. If their solicitations proved unsuccessful, their exertions were stimulated by the proprietor in person, who would sally forth from her den to aid the canvass, to admonish and to swear; and sometimes by the sentinel in charge, who assumed for the time being these functions of authority.

Women under like sad conditions, may still be observed in some of the principal streets of London, but I am happy to say a great improvement has taken place in this respect during the last twelve years. There still exist establishments in which the women live with their landlady, by whom they are provided with food, dress, and lodging, all which are charged to the women at an exorbitant price, and the landlady usually contrives to keep them in her debt; they have, however, the right of receiving and retaining their own money, and the privilege of accepting or declining, at their own discretion, the attentions offered by their visitors.

Houses in which Prostitutes Lodge. – I must now briefly notice the domiciliary arrangements of the various classes of independent prostitutes. These are so influenced – like our own homes – by the resources and taste of the individual, have so little local colour, and are besides so exceedingly well understood among men, that accurate pictures at any length would be as superfluous as fancy sketches would be out of place.

If we enter the house, or apartment, in a suburban neighbourhood – where, perhaps, the occupier of the shop below is non-resident – of the first-class prostitute, we find it neat or slovenly, plain or elegant, according to its mistress's income, the manners and tastes of her admirers, and her tendency to sobriety or the reverse. We have cheap and respectable lodgings, in reputable quarters of the town, wherein young and pleasing women of unambitious temperament will reside for years, receiving no visitors at home, anxiously guarding their characters there, and from choice involving themselves in no more sin than will serve to eke out their modest earnings, or provide a slender maintenance, which they may have been precluded from earning in their normal walk of life by the first false step. This numerous band, who, keenly alive to their painful position, willing to do better, unwilling – even for the sake of those wondrous magnets, dress and admiration – to join the ranks of the flashy and dissipated, are the proper objects of sympathy. London holds hundreds of them, not too far gone for true, permanent reform; and success would richly reward a far larger expenditure than can be expected at the hands of private charity.

These present us with the least degraded aspect of prostitution, but both in the western and eastern districts, especially in the latter, are to be found a great number of lodging-houses crowded together, in certain neighbourhoods of no fair fame, and called generically, in police reports, 'notorious brothels', devoted especially to the reception of prostitutes. They are clean or dirty – comparatively well or ill-furnished, according to the capital embarked in them. From houses in St John's Wood, Brompton, and Pimlico, to the atrocious slums of Blackfriars and Whitechapel, there are, of course, many steps, and with the rent at which the proprietors offer their apartments varies, of course, the style of the sub-tenants. In point of morality, there is, naturally, no difference; and in the general internal propriety, little enough. The most decently-minded woman who takes up her quarters in a circle of prostitutes, and, though she has a private apartment in which to receive visitors, betakes herself for society and distraction (as do always the inmates of such houses) to the common kitchen, must speedily fall to the common level. She finds that modesty and propriety are considered offensive hypocrisy. Liquor, in the intervals of business, is insisted upon by her companions and by the landlady, who makes a profit on the supply. Her company is sought for novelty's sake when she is a newcomer, and her absence or reserve is considered insulting when she is fairly settled; so, if she had any previous idea of keeping herself to herself, it is very soon dissipated. She finds, when she has no male visitors, a sort of communism established in her rooms, which she can only avoid by resorting to the common hall in the dirty kitchen. There is no making head against this practice in lodging-houses generally, and hence the remarkable uniformity in the habits, manners, dress, and demeanour of the three or four sub-sections of their inhabitants.

They are usually during the day, unless called upon by their followers, or employed in dressing, to be found, dishevelled, dirty, slipshod and dressing-gowned, in this kitchen, where the mistress keeps her *table-d'hôte*. Stupid from beer, or fractious from gin, they swear and chatter brainless stuff all day, about men and millinery, their own schemes and adventures, and the faults of others of the sisterhood. As a heap of rubbish will ferment, so surely will a number of unvirtuous women thus collected deteriorate, whatever their antecedents or good qualities previously to their being herded under the semi-tyranny of this kind of lodging-house. In such a household, all decency, modesty, propriety, and conscience must, to preserve harmony and republican equality, be planed down, and the woman hammered out, not by the practice of her profession or the company of men, but by association with her own sex and class, to the dead level of harlotry.

From such houses issue the greater number of the dressy females with whom the public are familiar as the frequenters of the Haymarket and the night-houses. Here they seem to rally, the last thing, from other parts of the town, when general society, and the most decent as well as lowest classes of prostitutes, are alike housed for the night. Here they throw the last allures of fascination to the prowler and the drunkard – hence wander to their lairs, disgusted and weary if alone – noisy and high-spirited if chance has lent them company.

To form an idea of the sort of life these women lead, we must listen to the evidence given at police courts. I extract the following from a leader in *The Times* for April 10, 1858, on evidence taken at the trial of an Italian, Giovanni Lani, who murdered one of these women for the sake of her jewelry:

> The house appears to have been well tenanted, and was, no doubt, a lucrative investment for Madame Levi's capital. 'Three or four women lodged in the house. They provided their own dresses and jewelry.' Madame Silvestre was one of these lodgers. She was not a *femme galante*, but still had a habit of walking the streets late at night. She lived in the front room of the second floor with her friend M. Théophile Mouton, by whose commercial profits she was supported. Madame Silvestre returned home on the night in question at one o'clock, and Héloise Thaubin, leaving the prisoner in her room, came down and had supper with her friend in the room where M. Mouton was in bed. About half-past two o'clock she went back to her own room, and at this seasonable hour Madame Silvestre, wishing for amusement, went up and borrowed a book from Héloise, which the prisoner, in his shirt,

handed out at the door. 'I then,' she says, 'went to bed, got up the next morning about twelve, and had breakfast at one.' Madame Silvestre, though not a *femme galante*, not only walked the streets, but was visited by male friends. 'When this occurred M. Mouton was generally out at his work.' This work M. Théophile Mouton tells us was the business of a commission agent. 'My business consists of selling every article that is intrusted to me. I have no offices, and never receive any business letters, because I am only a clerk, and have no business on my own account. I formerly used to deal in jewelry. The articles I sold were gilt or false jewelry.' Such is the account M. Mouton gives of his own professional pursuits. Besides these persons 'another man named Disher lived in the house. He carried on the business of a tailor. A woman lived with him who was called Mrs Disher'. Mr and Mrs Disher quarrelled on the night of the 23rd of February, and it was in consequence of the latter leaving her room and sitting on the stairs all night that she was able to hear the deceased's groans, and to recognize Lani as he came down laden with the murdered woman's spoils.

We have given this brief sketch of the house and its inmates, because No. 8, Arundel Court, was probably only a specimen of scores of other houses tenanted by this class of foreign adventuresses. They all seemed to have lived together with as little decency as brute animals. The last vestige of modesty which belongs even to the fallen seems to have been erased from the character of these cold, hard, money-grasping prostitutes and their paramours. They are well off, they wear their watches and chains and 'four rings on two fingers', they are 'proud of showing their jewelry', and they refuse 10 francs with disdain. The gentlemen lead an easy life. When the deceased's bedroom was broken open and her corpse found M. Théophile Mouton had not long returned home. 'He had been out for a walk with Mr Disher during the day, and he brought home something for dinner.' In short, we are introduced to a community which is existing in the most self-complacent manner on the wages of infamy, and in which each individual has the air of considering that he or she is doing nothing in the world to be ashamed of.

The keepers of the old dress houses were mostly females of extreme avarice, and often ferocious manners – the former sharpened by the unprincipled atmosphere in which they lived, and the latter by the necessity of preserving discipline among their tenants and dependents. They were ordinarily persons who had been bred to the business from youth, as relatives or old servants of their predecessors. Such an establishment was considered to be too lucrative to permit the idea of its dispersion upon the death or retirement of a proprietor; and as a matter of fact, the lease, goodwill, and stock-in-trade of a brothel were, in such an event, disposed of like those of any other lodging-house. Women who had been themselves kept or frequented by men of property were sometimes able to found or purchase one or more of them. A large share of their tenants' earnings passed through their hands, and a liberal portion always remained there. They were highly paid for liquors and eatables they procured on account of male visitors; and several instances are well authenticated of their having left ample means behind them, or having retired wealthy into private life. Things are, doubtless, changed.

It is to be feared, however, as we see, that there still exists a system analogous to that of woman farming, and resembling it only too closely, and that the dress house has merely given place to an institution too similar, viz., the dress lodging. Still the difference, though at first sight it may appear but one of name, is really one of degree. The dress girl was, as we have seen, the serf – the white slave of her proprietor, dependent on the latter for food and clothes and shelter, having no property of her own, or power over her own actions, but forced to fulfil the evil will of another by whom the fruits of her infamy were received. No property, no rights, no will, no hope – not one attribute, in short, of independent existence; the right alone remained to suffer and decay, while wretches more vile even than herself grew rich by her ruin. The dress lodger, like the dress girl, receives from the owner of the house in which she resides, clothes, and board and lodging, but the wages of her guilt are paid to herself. She obtains from the man whom she has enticed to the house as much money as she can, and the proprietor's interest in the booty amounts either to a part or the whole, according as her skill in extortion is small or great. Like the dress girl, she is exposed to the tender mercies of a brutal tyrant, who expects the surrender to herself of the gains of her corruption, but to her is, at least, conceded the acknowledgment of separate rights and independent existence.

Introducing Houses. – The establishments of certain procuresses . . . vulgarly called 'introducing houses', . . . are worth notice as the

43

leading centres of the more select circles of prostitution here. Unobtrusive, and dependent upon great exterior decency for a good connexion, they concern us as little from a sanitary as from a police point of view, but are not without an influence upon the morals of the highest society. Their existence depends upon the co-operation and discretion of various subordinate accomplices, and on the patronage of some of the many wealthy, indolent, sensual men of London, who will pay any premium for assurance against social discredit and sanitary damage. Disease is therefore rarely traceable to such a source, and notoriety and scandal almost as seldom; although impolitic economy on the gentleman's part, or indiscreet bearing towards any of the characters among whom he cannot be a hero, will induce them occasionally to hunt him and his follies into daylight, as a warning to others, not against the lusts of the flesh, but against sentiments which horse-leeches might consider illiberal. He usually obtains for his money security, comfort, and a superior class of prostitute, who is, according to his knowledge of the world or desires, presented to him as maid, wife, or widow – British, or imported direct from foreign parts. The female obtains fairly liberal terms, either directly from the paramour, or from the *entrepreneuse* (who, of course, takes good care of herself), the company of gentlemen, and, when this is an object with her, unquestionable privacy. A number of the first-class prostitutes have relations with these houses, and are sent for as occasion and demand may arise. I have heard of one establishment at which no female is welcome who has not some particular accomplishment, as music or singing. I am told these establishments are much more common in New York than in London.

A stranger might be long in London . . . without hearing of, and still longer without gaining access to, this aristocracy of brothels. Their frequenters are often elderly, sometimes married, and generally men of exclusive sets, upon whom it would not be to the proprietor's interest to impose even unseen association with the stranger or the *roturier* [commoner]. The leading persons in this line of business, who keep up regular relations with certain men of fashion, and sometimes means, make known to their clients their novel and attractive wares, one might almost say, by circular. A. finds a note at his club, telling him that a charming arrival, *de la plus grande fraîcheur* [in the absolute bloom of youth], is on view at Madame de L.'s. If he has no vacancy for a connexion, he may answer that a mutual friend, C., a very proper man, will call on such and such a day in —— road, or that Madame —— may drive the object round to his rooms at such another time; but that he has no great fancy at present for anything but a thoroughly warranted – in fact, an all-but modest – person. All parties handle the affair with mock refinement. Sometimes money passes direct, as third persons have to be arranged with; at others, the broker, or procuress, ventures her capital, and leaves recompense to the honour of her friends – some of whom, of course, fleece her, others do what is considered fair, and now and then may be so generous that she is, on the whole, perhaps, better off than if she traded on strict cash principles only. The pungent anecdotes which occur to me respecting such houses and their frequenters, would, if properly disguised, go little way in proof of their existence – which, by the way, must be patent enough to those who habitually read law reports – and as their unvarnished recital here would give my pages an air of levity quite foreign to my intentions, I must suppress them, and request the reader to take for granted, for the purpose of this survey, the existence of these superior haunts of London prostitution.

Accommodation Houses. – Accommodation houses for casual use only, the *maisons de passe* [houses of call] of London, wherein permanent lodgers are not received, are diffused throughout the capital; neither its wealth nor poverty exempting a district from their presence. I have not, and I believe that no other person has, any guide to their numbers or classification. I have seen various numerical estimates of these and other houses in print, some of them professing to be from public sources; but I attach in this respect little value to even those I have obtained from the police, as their framers seem neither to have settled for themselves or for the public the precise meanings of terms they employ. In the restricted sense in which I have employed the words 'accommodation house', I believe their number is limited. Few persons to whom I have spoken are now aware of more than four or five within two or three west end parishes, and as they almost invariably name the same, I am strengthened in my opinion that these lupanaria[18] are few. It were more desirable, indeed, that they should multiply than either class of the brothel proper above described; or that clandestine prostitution should be largely carried on in houses devoted to legitimate trades, and inhabited presumedly by modest females. The thorough elasticity of prostitution is shown in this as well as other ways; that there being a demand for more numerous and dispersed places of transient accommodation than at present exists, within the last few years numerous coffee-houses and legitimate taverns, at which in former days no casual lodgers would have been admitted, without scrutiny, now give accommodation of the kind, for the part openly, or when not exactly so, on exhibition of a slight apology for travelling baggage. This appears very clearly from the return for 1868, in which, for the first time, these houses are noticed, and in which they reach the important figure of 229. In addition to these coffee-shops, there are many restaurants at which people can obtain private rooms by ordering refreshments. Many abandoned women also are occupiers of houses, and though they do not receive lodgers, will, for a consideration and by arrangement, permit their rooms to be made use of by other women for immoral purposes. They naturally have a large acquaintance among prostitutes of their own class, so that it may be reasonably supposed that a large amount of illicit intercourse is in this way carried on; at the same time these houses are so quietly kept, that police supervision is, as regards them, impossible. The number of houses in the occupation of prostitutes has, it is true, materially decreased of late years, but is still considerable, Pimlico being the chief centre around which these women congregate. Formerly accommodation houses abounded, and were to be found in all parts of the town, some streets being entirely filled with them. Among others, I may mention Oxendon Street, close to the Haymarket; the front doors of the houses in this street were habitually left half open. King's Court was another locale in which several houses had existed from time immemorial; the narrow thoroughfare of Wych Street had also acquired an evil notoriety, the houses in this street, though ostensibly shops, being in reality all used for purposes of prostitution. Parish prosecutions have achieved the closing of most of these dens of iniquity, and the police returns show that the number of such houses throughout the metropolis has decreased to 132, against 649 in 1857, and 848 in 1841.

The few accommodation houses of London are generally thronged with custom, and their proprietors are of the same order as, and perhaps make even more money than, those of the lodging-houses. Their tariffs are various, and the accommodation afforded ranges between luxury and the squalor of those ambiguous dens, half brothel and half lodging-house, whose inhabitants pay their two-pences nightly. I believe that disorder is rarely encountered or courted by any casual frequenters of such places, and that in all of them but the vilest of the vile, the proprietors would be for their own sakes the last to countenance it, and the first to call in the aid of the law. This prosecution by parishes has had the effect of increasing the expense of using such of these houses as still exist. At the date of the introduction of the former edition of this work, the average sum charged for the hire of a room was about five shillings, but now the sum exacted for similar accommodation is never less than ten shillings, in the West End of London. In the East End and over the water,[19] the numbers and the tariff remain as small as they were twelve years ago.

PLEASURE GARDENS AND DANCING ROOMS

The Garden at Cremorne.[20] – It might seem rather late in the day to argue, on the grounds of its entertaining prostitutes among others, against the most beautiful public garden London can boast for the amusement of her people, and which, like many others of its kind, has taken, despite of strong objections, a position among the *faits accomplis* of the age. The union of Terpsichore and Melpomene,[21] long forbidden by puritanism, has now for some time been sanc-tioned by the magistracy; large capital has been invested in provid-ing local habitations for the young couple, and these are frequented without risk of more than nominal damage by great crowds of both sexes, all ranks, and all ages. No less than fifteen thousand people have been known to be present at Cremorne, on the occasion of the manager's benefit, and the nightly visitors during the fine season amount to between 1,500 and 2,000. As my present business, how-ever, is with the demeanour of London prostitution, I must unwillingly limit myself to the consideration of public out-door amusements, with reference to that common feature only, and state some impressions of travel on a pleasant July evening from Charing Cross to Chelsea.

As calico and merry respectability tailed off eastward by penny steamers, the setting sun brought westward hansoms freighted with demure immorality in silk and fine linen. By about ten o'clock, age and innocence, of whom there had been much in the place that day, had seemingly all retired, weary with a long and paid bill of amusements, leaving the massive elms, the grass-plots, and the geranium-beds, the kiosks, temples, 'monster platforms', and 'crystal circle' of Cremorne to flicker in the thousand gas-lights there for the gratification of the dancing public only. On and around that platform waltzed, strolled, and fed some thousand souls – perhaps seven hundred of them men of the upper and middle class, the remainder prostitutes more or less *prononcées*. I suppose that a hundred couples (partly old acquaintances, partly improvised) were engaged in dancing and other amusements, and the rest of the society, myself included, circulated listlessly about the garden, and enjoyed in a grim kind of way the 'selection' from some favourite opera and the cool night-breeze from the river.

The extent of disillusion he has purchased in this world comes forcibly home to the middle-aged man who in such a scene attempts to fathom former faith and ancient joys, and perhaps even vainly to fancy he might by some possibility begin again. I saw scores, nay hundreds, about me in the same position as myself. We were there – and some of us, I feel sure, hardly knew why – but being there, and it being obviously impossible to enjoy the place after the manner of youth, it was necessary, I suppose, to chew the cud of sweet and bitter fancies; and then so little pleasure came, that the Britannic solidity waxed solider than ever even in a garden full of music and dancing, and so an almost mute procession, not of joyous revellers, but thoughtful, care-worn men and women, paced round and round the platform as on a horizontal treadmill. There was now and then a bare recognition between passers-by – they seemed to touch and go, like ants in the hurry of business. I do not imagine for a moment they could have been aware that a self-appointed inspector was among them, but had they known it never so well, the intercourse of the sexes could hardly have been more reserved – *as a general rule*, be it always understood. For my part, I was occupied, when the first chill of change was shaken off, in quest of noise, disorder, debauchery, and bad manners. Hopeless task! The picnic at Burnham Beeches, that showed no more life and merriment than Cremorne on the night and time above-mentioned, would be a failure indeed, unless the company were antiquarians or undertakers. A jolly burst of laughter now and then came bounding through the crowd that fringed the dancing-floor and roved about the adjacent sheds in search of company; but that gone by, you heard very plainly the sigh of the poplar, the surging gossip of the tulip-tree, and the plash of the little embowered fountain that served two plaster children for an endless shower-bath. The *gratus puellae risus* [pleasing laughter of a girl] was put in a corner with a vengeance, under a colder shade than that of chastity itself, and the function of the very band appeared to be to drown not noise, but stillness.

The younger portion of the company formed the dances, and enjoyed themselves after the manner of youth, but I may fairly say, without offence to the most fastidious eye or ear. . . . The officiating member of the executive, Policeman T., had taken up an amiably discreet position, where his presence could in no way appear symptomatic of pressure, and the chances seemed to be, that had he stood so posed until his interference was necessary on behalf of public order, he might have been there to this day.

Lemonade and sherry seemed to please the dancers, and the loungers indulged the waiters' importunity with a rare order for bitter-beer. A strongish party of undergraduates in drinking – all males – were deepening their native dullness in a corner with bottled stout, and more seasoned vessels struggled against depression with hot grog. In front of the liquor-bar, called, in the language of the billographer, 'the gastronomic department', two rosy capitalists (their wives at Brighton or elsewhere) were pouring, for mere distraction's sake, libations of fictitious Möet, to the memory of auld lang syne with some fat old *dames de maison*, possibly extinct planets of the Georgian era. There was no drunkenness here to take hold of. As I have before recorded, there was among the general company barely vivacity, much less boisterous disorder. Let me try the assembly for immodest, brazen-faced solicitation by women. I declare my belief that I never saw the notoriously anti-sociable habit of English people more rigorously adhered to. Of the character of the female visitors – let me always say *with some exceptions* – I could have little moral doubt, but it was clear enough that self-proclamation by any great number of them was out of the question. It was open to the male visitors to invite attention and solicit acquaintance. No gentlemanly proposition of the kind would have been rebuffed, no courteous offer of refreshment, possibly, declined, but I am firmly of opinion, that had the most eligible men present tarried in hopes of overtures from the other side, they might have been there yet, with Policeman T.

As to the costumes of the company I have little more to say, than that pretty and quiet dressing was almost universal, and painted cheeks a rarity; but one or two physical characteristics seem worth mentioning. I saw many an etiolated eye and blanched chlorotic complexion, due to want of sun and air, and general defibrinization, but not more noticeable here than in Mayfair.[22] There was here and there a deplorable hectic flush, distinguishable enough from carmine; and I noticed a great prevalence of sunken eyes, drawn features, and thin lips, resulting from that absorption of the cellular tissue which leaves mere threads of muscle stretched upon the skull. Inasmuch as within my recollection women of the town had a well-known tendency to stoutness, and they now live no worse than heretofore, I am inclined to attribute these symptoms not so much (as is the vulgar error) to the practice of prostitution, as to the dancing mania, which has been the only remarkable change of late years in their mode of life, superadded in many instances to the action of early privations, and perhaps hard work in domestic service and millinery factories, upon naturally delicate or defective organizations.

There are other pleasure gardens in or about the London district, such as the gardens at North Woolwich, Highbury Barn, and Rosherville, but they do not call for any special notice, as, except that their frequenters are drawn chiefly from a lower class, they differ in no material respect from Cremorne.[23]

The principal dancing rooms of London are the two casinos known respectively as the Argyll Rooms and the Holborn.[24] Formerly there was a striking difference between these two places, the one receiving the upper, the other the under, current of the fast life of London; now, however, there is little of this distinction noticeable, and the visitor in quest, not of amusement, but of information, may feel assured that a visit to one is for all practical purposes a visit to both. They are open for music and dancing every evening, except Sunday, from half-past eight o'clock to twelve. The visitor, on passing the doors, finds himself in a spacious room, the fittings of which are of the most costly description, while brilliant gas illuminations, reflected by numerous mirrors, impart a fairy-like aspect to the scene. The company is, of course, mixed. Many of the men resorting to such places seek no doubt the opportunity of indulging their vicious propensities; but the majority of the better class go merely to while away an idle hour, because, unblessed by home ties, and weary of the cold monotony of their club, they find it pleasant to consume the '*post-prandial* weed' in some place where, while chatting with friends, they can hear good music and see pretty faces. The women are of course all prostitutes. They are for the most part pretty, and quietly, though expensively dressed, while delicate complexions, unaccompanied by the pallor of ill-health, are neither few nor far between. This appearance is doubtless due in many cases to the artistic manner of the make-up by powder and cosmetics, on the employment of which extreme care is bestowed. Few of these women, probably, could write a decent letter, though some might be able to play a little on the piano, or to sing a simple song. Their behaviour is usually quiet, little solicitation is observable, and all the outward proprieties of demeanour and gesture are strictly observed.

The proprietor, indeed, is careful to maintain the appearance, at least, of decorum among his visitors. Should any woman misconduct herself, she is pointed out to the door-keepers, with instructions not to admit her again to the rooms. No punishment could be heavier, no sentence more rigorously carried out. She will attempt in vain by disguise to avoid recognition, or by bribes to soften the watchful janitor. Her efforts will be met with some such rebuke as this: 'It's no use trying it on, Miss Polly; the gov'nor says you are not to go in, and, of course, you can't!' Her only chance of obtaining remission of the sentence is to induce some friend to plead with the proprietor on her behalf, who may, but does not always, readmit her after an exile of three months, and on her promising to behave herself in the strictest manner for the future.

On the whole, judging of the women who frequent these rooms by their dress, deportment, and general appearance, the visitor might be inclined to suppose them to belong to the kept mistress rather than the prostitute class. This is, however, not the case, as, with a few exceptions, they fall within the latter denomination. Many of them, no doubt, have a friend who visits them regularly, and who makes them a fixed allowance, not sufficient to keep them altogether, but substantial enough to make them careful in selecting their customers, and careful about accepting the company of a man in any way objectionable. This arrangement is perfectly understood by the 'friend' who pays his periodical visits, and to whom, of course, the woman is always at home. The sum expected by one of these women in return for her favours is about two or three sovereigns. Many will expect those who desire their company to stand them refreshment without stint, not only at the casino, but at some house of call later on in the night, suggesting champagne or 'phiz' as agreeable to their palate, and will be indisposed to return home until they have had their full evening's amusement. One woman merits a passing notice here, who has achieved a sudden notoriety, and given to the casino (previously to her appearance at it the least fashionable) a pre-eminence over its rival. There she holds a mimic court, attired unlike the rest of the frequenters, who come in their bonnets in full ball dress. She is surrounded by a crowd of admirers, idlers, and would-be imitators, and gives the tone to the establishment that she patronizes. It is said that the diamonds worn by this woman are worth £5,000. She is supplied daily from a florist in Covent Garden with a bouquet of the choicest flowers, amid which are interspersed specimens of the most beautifully coloured beetles, the cost being about 30s., and her habit on entering the rooms is to present this really splendid trifle to the female attendant at the wine bar, as a mark of her condescension and favour. On permission to visit her being requested, she would probably, like another celebrated 'fille de joie', take out her pocket-book and, after a careless glance at it, reply that she was full of engagements, but that if the petitioner would call at her house at a given hour that day week, she would, perhaps, spare him some twenty minutes of her society, for which favour she might expect the modest sum of £25.

The casinos, music-halls, and similar places are closed at twelve o'clock; after that hour the search for dissipation must be extended to other places, and loose persons of both sexes may be found congregated in the divans and night houses situate in the Haymarket* and adjoining streets. These places are for the most part small, ill-ventilated rooms, at which wine and other liquor, and also solid refreshment, can be procured. Here there is no amusement except such as the visitors can provide for themselves. Much of the restraint on the part of the women observable at the other places to which I

* [For a description of the Haymarket in 1857, see Appendix A, pp. 218–20].

have referred is, therefore, laid aside, and a very general *abandon* in conversation and behaviour on the part both of men and women is freely indulged in, while the opportunity of soliciting custom is certainly not neglected. The early closing bill gave a blow to these places, from which, notwithstanding the present unsatisfactory state of the law, they have not recovered; they are, however, neither so numerous nor so much frequented now as they were a few years ago.

Fast life in London has greatly changed during the last thirty years. It was the fashion formerly for those wishing to see life, as it is called, to go to the Theatre Royal, and between the acts to stroll into the saloons, and there look at the stout, over-dressed women who frequented these places, and resided in houses of ill-fame in the neighbouring slums. It was the correct thing to be taken after the theatre to Mother H.'s, and then to go to the 'Finish', having previously visited the notorious saloon in Piccadilly. From all these dens the police were excluded, and scenes were enacted very different from those now witnessed at the casinos.

Some shades of prostitution unknown to the more fashionable West are to be discerned in the East End of London. To acquaint myself with these, I made a pilgrimage in company with Captain Harris, Assistant Commissioner of Police, to the notorious Ratcliffe Highway.[25] We were attended by the Superintendent of the Executive Branch of the Metropolitan police, and two Inspectors. The night being very wet, the streets were comparatively empty, and therefore I can say little or nothing from personal observation about the condition of street prostitution in this district. I understand that it in no respect differs from what we see elsewhere. The first house we entered was one in which prostitutes reside. It was kept by a dark, swarthy, crisp-haired Jewess, half creole in appearance, who stated that she was a widow, and that having married a Christian, she had been discarded by her own people. To my inquiry whether she knew of many Jewesses who led a life of prostitution, she replied in the negative, giving as a reason that the Jews look after their people better than Christians, and assist them when in distress. The police Inspectors corroborated her statement, which seems to contradict the prevalent notion that houses of ill-fame are frequently kept by Jewesses. We went upstairs, and saw the rooms, eight in number, which were let out to as many women. The landlady told us that they pay 2*s*. when they bring home a visitor, and she thought that on an average they are lucky when they bring two each in the course of the evening. This woman was clearly indisposed to let us into her secrets, seeing us accompanied by the Inspectors, and entered into a rambling statement as to the care and leniency with which she treated her lodgers when they were 'out of luck'. She asserted, and the statement was corroborated by the girls, that they kept themselves; two may chum, or sleep together, when disengaged; but they receive the money they earn, and are not farmed out. The utmost pressure put upon them is, perhaps, that they are induced to go out and persevere in prostitution when otherwise indisposed to do so. When ill, they apply to the hospital, and St Bartholomew's appeared to be the favourite establishment. This house may be taken as a fair sample of the brothels existing in the East End of London.

The Inspectors next introduced us into a long, dirty room, behind a public-house. In the distance was a German band, such as one often sees in the streets. Several couples were waltzing, and other visitors were arranged round the room, smoking long pipes and drinking beer. We were next ushered into a large music-hall connected with a public-house. On the stage some interesting drama was going on, while the spectators drank and smoked; the majority were men, but they were in many instances accompanied by their wives and sweethearts. To make observations on the latter was my object, and I noted that in and out of the passages and bar were passing crowds of well-dressed women, according to East End fashions; some were prostitutes, but many were married women, according to the belief of my informants. This curious amalgamation – this elbowing of vice and virtue – constituted a very striking feature, and was to me a novel one. It is brought about, I presume, by the modern plan of these public-house amusements, enabling the mechanic, his wife and his daughters, to rationally spend the evening, as it is called, in witnessing plays, hearing music, and seeing dancing, at the same time that the man can smoke his pipe and drink his beer by the side of his wife. The landlords – two brothers, Jews, who told us they had been in Australia – assured us that they took the greatest pains to maintain order and decorum. My chief interest lay in considering the effect produced upon married women by becoming accustomed at these *réunions* to witness the vicious and profligate sisterhood flaunting it gaily, or 'first-rate', in their language – accepting all the attentions of men, freely plied with liquor, sitting in the best places, dressed far above their station, with plenty of money to spend, and denying themselves no amusement or enjoyment, encumbered with no domestic ties, and burdened with no children. Whatever the purport of the drama might have been, this actual superiority of a loose life could not have escaped the attention of the quick-witted sex.

What the result may be remains to be seen, but the enormous increase of establishments similar to the above must, I think, tend to the spread of immorality both in the East and West End of London. One explanation that I have received of the phenomenon, and it seems to me a plausible one, is that it is not unusual for the mechanic's wife to have sisters who are frail, and to these are accorded the greatest measure of kindness, and a sort of commiseration, which not infrequently culminates in their having a 'drop o' gin' together, and so forgetting for a time their mutual troubles – for the mechanic and the mechanic's wife have their troubles, and very serious ones, in providing for their daily wants, and any persons connected with them whom they see well-dressed, and with money in their pockets, command a kind of respect, although the source from whence the means are obtained may be a disreputable one. This same mingling of vicious with presumably respectable women is also noticeable at the Alhambra[26] and other music-halls at the West End of London, and in this respect they seem to me to exercise a more evil influence on the public morals than the casino, as to these last the notoriously profligate only resort.

It would be an endless task to examine into the features exhibited by prostitution in the different provincial towns throughout the kingdom. There may be slight differences in details, but the broad features are identical with those already presented to us in the Metropolis. Two places there are exceptionally circumstanced, and in them some special features will be looked for. Oxford and Cambridge have, through their Universities, one great cause of prostitution, viz., the presence in their midst of a floating population of unmarried males. Owing, however, to the restraints on indulgence imposed by university discipline, the amount of local prostitution is but little, if at all, in excess of the usual average of towns of similar dimensions, and it presents no features specially worthy of notice. I may, therefore, now pass on to another place where a large floating population of unmarried males is present, but the inducements to restraint above mentioned are absent.

With the sanction of Sir Richard Mayne, and with an introduction to Dr Barr, I made a visit to the camp and town of Aldershot to witness for myself the condition of prostitution at this great military centre, and to inquire on the spot into the state of things existing at the present day under the operation of the Contagious Diseases Act, which was applied to this district in April 1867, though periodical examinations were not instituted until April 1868. We were assisted in our investigations by Police Inspector Smith, whom I found a most useful cicerone in making my rounds in corners and places that it would have been impossible to see or venture into without his support. There appears to exist a sort of tacit understanding between these women and the authorities that they shall be suffered to pursue their calling unmolested so long as they abstain from acts of flagrant indecency. Neither is there here any third party to make a traffic of their bodies, and grow rich on the wages of their guilt. The prostitute is free to exercise her calling, and to receive the profits of it for herself. She obtains lodgings at the rate of about 3s. 6d. a week, payable *die in diem* [daily], for the daily accruing quota of which the landlord calls upon her every morning. One of these lodgings into which I was introduced by the inspector may be taken as a fair specimen of the class. It was a small room on the first floor of a cottage, approached by a steep narrow staircase, furnished in the most primitive manner, containing only a bed with the usual covering, one or two rough chairs, and the other commonest necessaries of a bedroom. Only one condition beyond punctual payment of the rent is attached to the tenancy. The landlord is usually the proprietor of a beer-house or some other place of public entertainment, which the lodger must patronize during her stay. She is required to spend her evenings there until the tattoo sounds at 9.30, after which hour she is free to go where she pleases. She is also expected to aid the landlord in the sale of liquor, both by inducing the soldiers to drink, and by accepting whatever drink may be offered to her by them. Most of the girls have or acquire a habit of drinking: some few abstain, and while accepting, find means to avoid partaking of the refreshment offered to them. They are sneered at by their more debased companions, but are distinguished by their superior dress, and greater neatness, spending, in fact, in this manner the money that they would otherwise squander, like their companions, in the beer-houses. There is at Aldershot no street prostitution permitted; the woman's hunting grounds are the above-named public rooms.

The daily gains are not large. The generous and prodigal son of Mars who has lately received his pay or his loot money will, perhaps, bestow half a crown in return for the favours granted to him, but the usual honorarium is 1s. For this poor pay, these wretched women are content to surrender their persons. To obtain a subsistence, a woman must take home with her about eight or ten lovers every evening, returning to her haunts after each labour of love . . . to dance or drink beer until a fresh invitation to retire is received by her. As night approaches, each woman usually seeks her room, carrying with her ale or other stimulating liquor, which she shares with her fellow-lodgers, and wakes in the morning languid from the night's debauch to breakfast off beefsteaks and beer. Thus are her vile earnings grossly squandered, with nothing saved for an evil day. For help when her own resources fail her, she depends on the contributions of those of her companions whom chance has for the time being more befriended; and in justice to these women, it must be said that they are always ready to afford each other this mutual assistance.

I visited with the inspector the different public rooms, which were crowded with soldiers and women. To my surprise I saw no instance of drunkenness, no riot or romping, and heard no indecent jests or songs. This propriety of conduct may have been due to the word having been passed that the inspector was making his rounds with the two doctors; if drunkenness or other disorderly conduct had been indulged in previously to our arrival, traces of it would, I should think, have remained. The lodgings before referred to are attached, or at least contiguous, to the public rooms owned by the different landlords. They naturally do not afford sufficient accommodation for the vast mass of Aldershot prostitution. Many of the women, therefore, live in lodgings in the town, and as these apartments are at a considerable distance from the soldiers' haunts, they take their temporary companions to rooms in their immediate neighbourhood that can be hired for a short time for this purpose.

We entered one of these dens. In a room, opening on to a court, reached by a dirty street, and looking more like an old rag and bottle shop than anything else, sat an old man, huddled close up to the fire, surrounded by candlesticks ready for use, while in a trussel bed, covered up with shawls and flannel, and propped up by pillows, sat a woman, who must have been in her day remarkably handsome, but on whom the hand of disease lay heavily. She had been an out-patient at the Brompton Consumption Hospital, and had obtained some relief there, but her complaint being incurable, she returned home, though the bleak air of Aldershot did not agree with her; and truly as she lay there coughing and wheezing and grumbling, she seemed a doomed being, whose life was not worth a week's purchase. But what had these people to do with prostitution? All and everything! The inspector pointed out to me a range of cottages, with lights in their windows; each room contained a man and woman, and the cottages all belonged to this aged and decrepit couple. It seems that any woman desiring to use a room would come in for a candle to the old man, who, in a few minutes, would crawl furtively to get his twopence for the use of the room, which he would bring back to the old woman lying at the receipt of custom, as above described. The daughter of this precious pair was, at the time of my visit, in the hospital, under treatment. She hires a room of her parents, paying them the rent every morning, and is as noted a prostitute as any other wretched frequenter of her father's miserable rooms. In a house of a similar nature that we visited, we found the landlady engaged in washing, with her two little children lying in bed asleep, with the happy smile of childhood on their faces, unconscious of the surrounding depravity, while two boys scarcely in their teens were employed to collect the twopences from their parents' customers. Thus is it that some, at least, of our population are brought up, and a constant supply maintained of recruits for the dangerous classes.

Having now surveyed the extent of prostitution, together with the more salient points connected with the life and habits of its victims, it will not be without profit to consider attentively, and at some length, the condition to which these unhappy women are reduced, paying especial regard to two points of considerable importance: ... whether the effects produced are permanent; and how far the facts ascertained with regard to prostitution bear out the notions generally prevailing on this subject.

When the licentious epoch of the Restoration, due itself to the national recoil from the abortive attempt of the Puritans to enact religion and morality, was succeeded by the austerity of the Roman Catholic James and the decorous court of William and Mary, and while the fixed and floating population of the capital was increasing with the facilities of travel, the growth of trade, and the general wealth, there is no doubt that long rampant immorality – incurable at short notice – was but held repressed, and compelled to hide its head. A remarkable impetus was therefore given to comparatively secret prostitution, corresponding to the decrease in adultery and overt concubinage which about that time ceased to be indispensable qualifications of the man of parts and fashion.

When I consider that genteel society was passing during the period of the Augustan essayists from a political and moral delirium towards a state of repose, and the artificial scarcity of trained intellects which yet recent events had created among the class for whom they wrote – I am not surprised that earnest authors, careful of administering strong meat to babes, should have elected to work upon the public mind, as they did, with types and parables. But I do wonder that so many able men, from that period to our own day, who might have touched moral pitch without the fear or imputation of defilement, have, whether through moral cowardice or considerations of expediency, still as it were by concert, been content to do little more than retouch and restore the pictures of the ancient masters, adding, from time to time, perhaps, some horrid feature. Thus has been painfully built up a sort of 'bogie' in a corner cupboard, unheeded by the infant, terrible to the aged, the untempted, and others whom it concerned not; while the flower of the people have rushed into the streets and worshipped the immodest Venus.

Thus, I believe, was firmly rooted – if it did not thus originate – and thus has mightily prospered, remaining even to our day an overshadowing article of almost religious belief, the notion that the career of the woman who once quits the pinnacle of virtue involves the very swift decline and ultimate total loss of health, modesty, and temporal prosperity. And herein are contained three vulgar errors:

1. That once a harlot, always a harlot.

2. That there is no possible advance, moral or physical, in the condition of the actual prostitute.

3. That the harlot's progress is short and rapid.

And the sooner fearless common sense has cleared the ground of fallacy, the sooner may statesmen see their way to handle a question of which they have not denied the importance.

It is a little too absurd to tell us that 'the dirty, intoxicated slattern, in tawdry finery and an inch thick in paint' – long a conventional symbol of prostitution – is a correct figure in the middle of the nineteenth century. If she is not apocryphal, one must at least go out of the beaten path to find her. She is met with, it is true, in filthy taps, resorts of crime, and in the squalid lairs of poverty – rarely courting the light, but lurking in covert spots to catch the reckless, the besotted, and the young of the opposite sex. And though such may be even numbered by hundreds, it must, on reflection, be conceded by those who have walked through the world with open eyes, that, considering the square mileage of the Metropolis, and the enormous aggregate I am treating of, they are but as drops in an ocean. The Gorgon of the present day against whom we should arm our children should be a woman who, whether sound or diseased, is generally pretty and elegant – oftener painted by Nature than by art – whose predecessors cast away the custom of drunkenness when the gentlemen of England did the same – and on whose backs, as if following the poet's direction, *in corpore vili* [on the vile body], the ministers of fashion exhibit the results of their most egregious experiments.

The shades of London prostitution . . . are as numberless as those of society at large, and may be said to blend at their edges, but no further. The microcosm, in fact, exhibits, like its archetype, saving one, all the virtues and good qualities, as well as all the vices, weaknesses, and follies.

The great substitution of unchastity for female honour has run through and dislocated all the system; but it must not be imagined that, though disordered and for a time lost to our sight, the other strata of the woman's nature have ceased to exist.

The class maintain their notions of caste and quality with all the pertinacity of their betters. The greatest amount of income procurable with the least amount of exertion, is with them, as with society, the grand gauge of position; and each individual, like her betters, sets up for private contemplation some ideal standard with which she may compare, deeming most indispensable to beauty and gentility the particular elements she may best lay claim to.

* * *

The order may be divided into three classes – the 'kept woman' (a repulsive term, for which I have in vain sought an English substitute), who has in truth, or pretends to have, but one paramour, with whom she, in some cases, resides; the common prostitute, who is at the service, with slight reservation, of the first comer, and attempts no other means of life; and the woman whose prostitution is a subsidiary calling.

The presence of the individual in either of these categories may of course depend upon a thousand accidents; but once in either rank, as a general rule her footing is permanent while her prostitution, in any sense of the word, continues. There is, although the moralist insist otherwise, little promotion, and less degradation. The cases of the latter are quite exceptional; those of the former less rare, but still not frequent. The seduction and primary desertion of each woman who afterwards becomes a prostitute is an affair apart; and the liaison of a woman with her seducer is generally of the shortest. This over, her remaining in the ranks of honest society, or her adoption of prostitution, becomes her question. Some few voluntarily take the latter alternative. Domestic servants, and girls of decent family, are generally driven headlong to the streets for support of themselves and their babies; needlewomen of some classes by the incompatibility of infant nursing with the discipline of the workshop. Those who take work at home are fortunate enough, and generally too happy, to reconcile continuance of their labours with a mother's nursing duties, and by management retain a permanent connexion with the army of labour, adopting prostitution only when their slender wages become insufficient for their legitimate wants. . . .

Our first, or superior order, recruits its ranks as follows:

1. From women cohabiting with, or separately maintained by, their seducers.

2. From kept women who are, as it were, in the business, and transfer their allegiance from party to party at the dictates of caprice or financial expediency.

3. From women whom men select for a thousand and one reasons, from promiscuous orders – or, as commonly said, 'take off the town'.

4. From women similarly promoted from the *ouvrière* [working] class.

The prominent or retiring position the individual occupies in these three divisions – allowing, of course, for exceptions influenced by her idiosyncrasies – depends mainly upon gaiety or gravity of temperament. These characteristics exaggerated, on the one hand, into boisterous vulgarity, on the other, into nervous retirement – both chequered, more or less, at times, by extreme depression and hysterical mirth – pervade the devotees to this calling, and influence their whole career. A woman endowed with the one may, for a time, by force of circumstances, assume the other – but for a time only. The spring recoils, and the natural character asserts its sway. It is superfluous almost to allude, among men of the world, to the arrogant and offensive conduct into which some prostitutes of the upper class, and of mercurial temperament, will be betrayed, even when permitted to elbow respectability and good conduct in public places; or to their intense assumption of superiority over their less full-blown sisters, on the strength of an equipage, an opera box, a saddle-horse, a Brompton villa, and a visiting list. This is the kind of woman of whom I said just now that the loss of her honour seemed to have intensified every evil point in her character. She it is who inflicts the greatest scandal and damage upon society, and by whom, though she is but a fraction of her class, the whole are necessarily, but injudiciously, if not cruelly, judged. This is the flaunting, extravagant quean, who, young and fair – the milliners' herald of forthcoming fashions – will daily drag a boyish lover (for whose abject submission she will return tolerable constancy, and over whose virtue she presides like another Dian), [willy-nilly], like a lackey, in her train to Blackwall parties,[27] flower shows, and races – night after night to the 'select ballet balls', plays, or public dancing saloons – will see him gaily, along with jockeys who are no gentlemen and gentlemen who are all jockey, through his capital or his allowances, and then, without a sigh, enlist in the service of another – perhaps his intimate friend – till she has run the gauntlet as kept mistress through half a dozen short generations of men about town.

Descend a step to the promiscuous category, and trace the harlot to whom a tavern-bar was congenial instead of repulsive on her first appearance there – say at 16 or 18 years of age. At 30 and at 40 you will find her (if she rises in the scale) the loudest of the loud, in the utmost blaze of finery, looked on as 'first-rate company' by aspiring gents, surrounded by a knot of 'gentlemen' who applaud her rampant nonsense, and wondering, hotel-sick, country men of business, whose footsteps stray at night to where she keeps her foolish court.

She is a sort of whitewashed sepulchre, fair to the eye, but full of inner rottenness – a mercenary human tigress; albeit there exists at times some paltry bulldog, nursed in the same Bohemian den, who may light up all the fires of womanhood within her – some rascally enchanter, who may tame her at the height of her fury, when none else human may approach her, by whispering or blows. Exigeant of respect beyond belief, but insufferably rude, she is proud and high-minded in talk one moment, but not ashamed to beg for a shilling the next. The great sums of money she sometimes earns, she spends with romantic extravagance, on her toilette partly, and partly circulates, with thoughtless generosity, among the lodging-house sharks and other baser parasites that feed upon her order.

Should such a light-minded woman descend in the scale of promiscuous prostitution, which of course is a matter of possibility, though not so likely as her rise, she will still be found the same. As no access of fortune will do much towards humanizing, so no ill-luck will soften or chasten her. She will be in Lambeth or Whitechapel as I have described her in Soho or the Haymarket – a drunken, brawling reprobate – but in a lower orbit.

On the other hand, the sad career in prostitution of the softer-minded woman, in whatever rank she may be, will be marked and affected by that quality. Whatever befall her in this vale of tears, the gentle-minded woman will be gentle still; and with this native hue will be tinged all her dealings with the sisterhood, and with the rough rude males whom ever and anon it is her fate to meet. If fortunate enough to have the acquaintance of some quiet men of means, she will not be puffed up with vain-gloriousness, but seeking comfort in obscurity, and clinging fast to what respect she may gain of others, will profess – what I dare say she really often feels – disgust at brazen impudence, and all the pomps and vanities. Whether this eschewal be from real delicacy, or considerations of economy, or because any sort of notoriety, instead of cementing, as in the case of others mentioned, would be fatal to their particular liaison, it is hard to say; but, however that may be, it is no less true that hundreds of females so constituted are at this moment living within a few miles of Charing Cross, in easy if not elegant circumstances, with every regard to outward decorum and good taste, and shocking none of the public who will not attempt unnecessarily close investigation, but for all that 'in a state of prostitution'. The ease and comparative prosperity that inflates the lighter woman into a public nuisance have no such effect upon such a one as I have spoken of last. They but cause her to prize each day more highly peace and quietness – more sadly to regret the irrevocable past – more profoundly to yearn after some way out of the wilderness.

Among the promiscuous prostitutes of the milder order will be found a numerous band, who, unlike the magnificent virago of the supper-shops, rarely see the evening lamps. Sober, genteelly dressed, well ordered, often elegant in person – such girls have the taste and the power to select their acquaintances from among the most truly eligible men whom the present false state of society debars from marriage. Their attractions, indeed, are of the subdued order that neither the hot blood of the novice nor the prurient fancy of the used-up rake could appreciate. Of course, they take the chances of their calling. They know that a short acquaintance often turns their sorrow into joy, and opens out a better, happier future. They know, too, that one unlucky hour may make them scatterers of pestilence. What wonder, then, that woman's tact, sharpened by uses of adversity, should induce them to prefer the respect and counsel of well-bred men of settled character to the evanescent passion of mere youths. From the former they get lessons, rarely thrown away, on the value of repose and thrift; from the latter, only new proofs of folly and fickleness. With the one they may for a time forget their occupation; with the other, only sharpen memory. They exhibit at times the greatest respect for themselves, and for the opinions, scruples, and weaknesses of those with whom they are connected, and whom they love to call their 'friends'; and, above all, they are notable for the intensity of love with which they will cling to the sister, the mother, the brother – in fact, to any one 'from home' who, knowing of their fall, will not abjure them, or, ignorant of their present calling, still cherishes some respect and regard for them. The sick man is safe in their hands, and the fool's money also. There is many a tale well known of their nursing and watching, and more than will do so could tell of the harlot's guardianship in his hour of drunkenness. I have seen the fondest of daughters and mothers among them. I fancy that where they have that regard for men which they are too pleased to return for mere politeness, they are well-meaning, and not always foolish friends – no abettors of extravagance, and, so far as absolute honesty is concerned, implicitly to be relied on. They are more dupes than impostors – more sinned against than sinning – till the play is played out, the pilgrimage accomplished, and they who have long strained their eyes for a resting-place quit the painful road (as I say they mostly do) for a better life on earth; or, leaving hope behind on their discharge from the hospitals, issue to an obscurity more melancholy and degraded than ever. For of such on whom has fallen the lot of foul disease, or whom a loss of health or beauty has deprived of worthy associates, are the abject maundering creatures who haunt the lower dens of vice and crime. Deficient in mental and physical elasticity to resist the downward pressure of intermittent starvation and undying conscience, they are pulled from depth to lower deep, by men who trample, and women of their class who prey upon them. Liquor, which other organizations adopt as a jovial friend and partner of each gleam of sunshine, is to these the medicine and permanent aggravation of dejected misery. Cruelly injured by the other sex, they moodily resolve to let retribution take its course through their diseased agency; trodden underfoot by society, what can society expect from them but scorn for scorn?

The woman, the castle of whose modesty offered stoutest resistance to the storm of the seducer, often becomes in time the most abiding stronghold of vice. Saturated with misery and drink, perhaps then crime and disease, dead long in heart, and barely willing to live on in the flesh – ceasing to look upward, ceasing to strike outward, she will passively drift down the stream into that listless state of moral insensibility in which so many pass from this world into the presence of their Judge.

'And here' – I can fancy some reader interrupting – 'here ends your catechism. You have led us a painful pilgrimage through the obscurest corners behind the scenes of civilized society, casting, by the way, a glare on matters from whose contemplation mature refinement would gladly be spared, and the bare conception of which should be studiously shut out from youth and innocence. At the end of all you show us the heroine of your prurient sympathy overtaken by her doom. We have seen by turns reflected on your mirror the pampered concubine and the common street-walker – the haunts of dissipation and the foul ward; but you dissent from our religious, and at least venerably antique belief, that between these stages there is an organized progression. You cast your lantern ray at last upon a guilty, solitary wreck, perishing, covered with sores, in some back garret, in a filthy court; and you ask us to believe that this is not retribution.'

I do, in truth. For if this fate were general – inevitable, unless by direct intervention of Providence, or arrest of its decree by perverse interposition of science – I might admit the truth of my opponents' creed. But I maintain, on the contrary, that such an ending of the harlot's life is the altogether rare exception, not the general rule; that the downward progress and death of the prostitute in the absolute ranks of that occupation are exceptional also, and that she succumbs at last, not to that calling, nor to venereal disease, but in due time, and to the various maladies common to respectable humanity.

I hope to show fair grounds for these conclusions, and for my opinion that the doors of escape from this evil career are many; that those who have walked in it do eagerly rush through them, neither lingering nor looking behind; that the greatest and most flagrant are not stricken down in the pursuit of sin, nor does the blow fall when it might be of service as an example. If in the following pages I can do something towards this, it may be more justly argued, I think, that an all-wise, all-merciful God has provided these escapes, than that those whom fate overtakes within the vicious circle are selected by His design. And if so, it justly follows that those are less impious and erring, than furthering God's will, who would widen the gates of the fold of penitence and rest, gather by all possible means yet another crop to the harvest of souls, and claim the Christian's noble birthright of rejoicing over more and yet more repentant sinners.

To those who may ask, 'What can it matter to us what becomes of them? The subject may be statistically interesting, but no further. The interests of society demand that a disgusting inquiry should be discouraged, lest by chance the eyes of youth should be polluted' – I have this much to say. That the Utopian epoch being long since passed, if indeed it ever had a beginning, when the book of evil could be sealed to the people, it is time that the good and wise, not flinching from the moral pitch, should emulate the evil and the crooked-minded in their attempts to guide the public.

The streets of London are an open book, and very few may walk therein who cannot and will not inquire and read for themselves. Shall those who of right should be commentators for ever leave an open field to the bigoted and the sinful, with the idea of fostering a degree of purity to which the state of society precludes a more than fictitious existence? Shall dirt be allowed to accumulate, only because it is dirt?

A few stubborn figures may perhaps assist the candid reader towards, at least, a partial removal of impressions he may have received, in common with a large portion of the public, as to the causes of mortality among prostitutes.

Some years ago, in 1851, the Registrar-General, Major Graham,[28] with his usual politeness and at considerable trouble, extracted for me the number of deaths ascribable to venereal diseases which occurred in the Metropolis during the years 1846–48, and again in the year 1868. I am further indebted to him and Dr Farr for the additional tables, and from them I have compiled the following:

Table, distinguishing the Males from the Females, their Ages, and the Forms of the Disease of which they died in London

| | FEMALES | | | | | | MALES | | | | | | Male and Female aged 15–65 |
	15 to 25	25 to 35	35 to 45	45 to 55	55 to 65	Total aged 15–65	15 to 25	25 to 35	35 to 45	45 to 55	55 to 65	Total aged 15–65	
Syphilis	3	12	5	7	2	29	4	4	2		4	14	43
Phagedaenic disease[29]	2	3	—	—	—	5	2	—	—	—	—	2	7
Disease of bone	—	1	1	—	1	3	—	1	—	—	—	2	5
Ulceration of larynx ..	1	2	—	—	—	3	1	5	—	1	—	6	9
Venereal disease.. ..	—	3	1	—	—	4	1	2	—	—	—	3	7
Consumption	2	6	1	—	—	9	1	6	—	2	1	10	19
Chest affection	1	2	—	—	—	3	1	1	—	—	1	3	6
Paralysis	—	—	—	1	—	1	—	1	—	—	—	1	2
Cachexia[30] and debility	2	2	3	1	—	8	—	—	1	3	—	4	12
Erysipelas	5	1	2	—	—	8	3	5	1	—	—	9	17
All diseases..	16	32	13	9	3	73	13	25	4	6	6	54	127
Syphilis, in the three years, 1864, 1865, and 1866	35	37	24	11	4	111	15	25	20	11	7	78	189

The first thing that strikes the reader here is the paucity of fatal cases. Notwithstanding the frequency of the complaint in the Metropolis, . . . only 127 deaths are noted during 156 weeks, out of a population amounting to more than 3,000,000, or on the average less than one a week.

The above table, I think, disposes of the hypothesis that any large number of females, whether prostitutes or not, die annually of syphilis. It exhibits only 73 women to 54 men; and this proportion is more striking when we consider that the female population of London is to the male as 120 to 100, or six to five.

In order to corroborate my assertions made some years ago, that syphilis was not a fatal disease, I again applied, in May 1857, to

Deaths from Syphilis of Females at Different Ages in England and Wales, and in London, in the years 1855, 1866, and 1867

	England and Wales	London	England and Wales	London	England and Wales	London
	1855	*1855*	*1866*	*1866*	*1867*	*1867*
Under 1 year ..	269	54	556	166	582	170
1 year	28	4	43	4	38	9
2 years	11	—	9	3	6	1
3 years	7	—	4	3	3	—
4 years	3	1	3	—	2	—
Total under 5 years	318	59	615	176	631	180
5–10 years	5	—	4	1	1	—
10–15 years	4	1	1	—	1	—
15–20 years	16	2	13	7	7	2
20–25 years	18	3	39	10	42	6
25–30 years	25	2 }	57	12	68	13
30–35 years	25	3 }				
35–40 years	20	3 }	42	6	51	7
40–45 years	11	3 }				
45–50 years	13	1 }	20	5	26	2
50–55 years	5	— }				
55–60 years	4	1 }	9	1	10	1
60–65 years	3	— }				
65 years and upwards	1	—	9	1	3	1
Total, all ages ..	468	78	827	219	840	212

Major Graham, and he kindly forwarded me the annexed table, which is curious as showing how large a proportion of the female mortality from syphilis falls upon infants and children under five years of age.

In a letter, dated 1868, with which Dr Farr has favoured me, that gentleman says: 'It is probable that at least a portion of the increase in the number of cases of syphilis is due to improved and more accurate registration.'

Let persons who have been through the syphilitic wards of hospitals call to mind the stamp of women to be seen there. The fact of a girl's seduction generally warrants her possession of youth, health, good looks, and a well-proportioned frame – qualifications usually incompatible with a feeble constitution. She, at least, meets the world with power of resistance beyond the average of women in her station. Notwithstanding all her excesses (and legion is their name) the prostitute passes through the furnace of a dissipated career less worse from wear than her male associates; and when she withdraws from it – as withdraw she will in a few years, for old prostitutes are rarely met with – she is seldom found with her nose sunk in, her palate gone, or nodes upon her shins.

Nay, more, experience teaches that frequently the most violent and fatal cases among women take their rise during the period of comparative innocence, before their adoption of prostitution, and their consequent acquirement of worldly knowledge. I grieve to say that there are systematic seducers so unutterably base as not only to pollute the mind of modest girls, but simultaneously to steep their bodies in most lamentable corruption. Their want of knowledge and ingenuous sense of shame induce, in cases such as these, aggravation of suffering from which the experienced prostitute is comparatively exempt.

So rare is death from uncomplicated syphilis, that many a surgeon has never witnessed a single instance; and those attached to hospitals where venereal diseases are specially treated have so few opportunities of witnessing post-mortems of persons who have succumbed to them, that it becomes interesting to inquire how they produced death. This is answered by the return from the Registrar-General. In the first place, erysipelas may attack the sores of *all* patients entering a hospital, and a certain number of syphilitic patients, as of other classes, die from this cause. Syphilis, therefore, acted but a secondary part in producing the fatal termination of the 17 cases of erysipelas in the above table.

★ ★ ★

Syphilis is most frequently fatal when it has reached the tertiary form, in the neglected cases of which we observe its greatest ravages. Patients are destroyed by the deposit of bone, which, pressing on the brain, produces paralysis, convulsions, and other nervous phenomena. In other cases caries of bones takes place, and exhaustion causes death. Occasionally the cartilages of the larynx fall in, and the patient dies asphyxiated. Lastly, the hopeless and intense form of tertiary syphilis, known as syphilitic cachexia, sometimes comes on, and gradually leads to a fatal termination, as in the following instance.

I was called to see a young girl who was stated to be very ill, at King Street, Islington. I found my poor dispensary patient living in an attic, in one of the small streets off the Lower Road, attended by her mother, without fire or furniture, almost without clothing. She lay, doubled up in the corner of this bare room, on an old mattress stuffed with shavings, with no bed-linen but a thin patched quilt and a few rags. She was covered with rupia,[31] and attenuated to the last degree, though bearing marks of having been a very pretty girl.

She had never left her mother's roof for twenty-four hours; but had nevertheless been seduced, diseased, and deserted – sad and frequent story – and, as long as she was able, had in secret attended at a hospital. Her mother had never left her, and – so naïve had she remained in this city of licentiousness – was apparently unaware of the nature of her child's disorder. Never applying to the parish, she had obtained a bare subsistence by her needle, until her ministering office had shut out even this precarious support. She had parted with her every property, till, indeed, no warmth could be obtained except by creeping close together under their miserable counterpane.

At once, seeing the nature of the case, and the impossibility of my being of material service to this poor creature, I spoke of the hospital, but neither mother nor daughter would hear of it: they had never been separated, and never would be. Persuasion was in vain. Assistance was procured; still the debility increased, and I was absolutely obliged to threaten the interference of the parish officers. At last the patient consented to be carried to the hospital, but at such a stage of the complaint this could only be effected with the greatest difficulty. She was, however, admitted into St Bartholomew's, and the comforts which that noble institution so liberally furnishes to its sick, at first caused her to rally, but an immense abscess formed in her thigh, and she sank in a short time under syphilitic cachexia.

Who could have seen that hapless, unoffending victim to her woman's trust and man's barbarity, hurried to an early grave, without asking himself could such a one have been marked out for example and for punishment by a discerning Providence, as some would tell us? . . .

[Despite] the public and popular notion that by deaths in hospitals we rid ourselves of the immoral female population, . . . not a single female died from syphilis [at St Bartholomew's Hospital in 1868], although some of the worst cases are admitted to the wards, and the most accurate accounts are kept. . . .

Syphilis is the fate neither of the bulk, nor of an important fraction, of prostitutes. . . . To meet the hypothesis that, if such is not the fact, they may at least fall victims to suicide, intemperance, or complaints incidental to an irregular course of life, I have made special inquiries among the medical attendants of hospitals, penitentiaries, as well as well-informed private practitioners, and certain parish authorities. Their replies seem to corroborate my impressions that the combined operation of all these agencies, in addition to venereal complaints, is inadequate to extirpate, as alleged, a generation of prostitutes every few years, and that no other class of females is so free from general disease as this is. I find that in 1867, 83 females committed suicide; 7 of these were under 20 years of age; 76 were aged 20 and upwards. There was no reason to believe that even one-half were prostitutes.* . . .

The records of our civil courts have recently proved how hard it is to kill a person of fine constitution, supplied designedly with unlimited liquor and relays of pot companions; and we know again, that by the thorough prostitutes the sexual act is generally performed with the least possible exertion, and that her visitor is not uncommonly himself debauched and, for the time being, impotent. . . .

* It has been supposed that many prostitutes become insane. We find little evidence corroborative of this opinion. . . . It is a question whether grief, anxiety, and broken hours may not have a greater share in dethroning the reason than sensuality.

71

If we compare the prostitute at thirty-five with her sister, who perhaps is the married mother of a family, or has been a toiling slave for years in the over-heated laboratories of fashion, we shall seldom find that the constitutional ravages often thought to be necessary consequences of prostitution exceed those attributable to the cares of a family and the heart-wearing struggles of virtuous labour.

How then is the disparition of this class of women to be accounted for, as they are neither stricken down in the practice of harlotry, nor by their own hands, nor by intemperance and venereal disease, nor would seem to perish of supervening evils in any notable proportion? Do they fall by the wayside, as some assume, like leaves of autumn, unnoticed and unnumbered, to be heaped up and to rot? Do unknown graves conceal, not keeping green the lost one's memory, and the obscure fallible records of the pauper burials at last confound all clue and chance of tracing her? Is she filtered again into the world through a reformatory? or does she crawl from the sight of men and the haunts of her fellows to some old homely spot in time to linger and to die?

I have every reason to believe, that by far the larger number of women who have resorted to prostitution for a livelihood, return sooner or later to a more or less regular course of life. Before coming to this conclusion I have consulted many likely to be acquainted with their habits, and have founded my belief upon the following data. Whatever be the cause of a female becoming a prostitute, one thing is certain – before she has carried on the trade four years, she has fully comprehended her situation, its horrors and its difficulties, and is prepared to escape, should opportunity present itself. The constant humiliation of all, even of those in the greatest affluence, and the frequent pressure of want attendant on the vocation of the absolute street-walker, clouding the gaiety of the kept woman, and driving the wedge of bitter reflection into the intervals of the wildest harlot's frenzy, are the agencies which clear the ranks of all but veterans who seem to thrive in proportion to their age.

Incumbrances rarely attend the prostitute who flies from the horrors of her position. We must recollect that she has a healthy frame, an excellent constitution, and is in the vigour of life. During her career, she has obtained a knowledge of the world most probably above the situation she was born in. Her return to the hearth of her infancy is for obvious reasons a very rare occurrence. Is it surprising, then, that she should look to the chance of amalgamating with society at large, and make a dash at respectability by a marriage? Thus, to a most surprising, and year by year increasing extent, the better inclined class of prostitutes become the wedded wives of men in every grade of society, from the peerage to the stable, and as they are frequently barren, or have but a few children, there is reason to believe they often live in ease unknown to many women who have never strayed, and on whose unvitiated organization matrimony has entailed the burden of families.

Others who, as often happens, have been enabled to lay by variable sums of money, work their own reclamation as established milliners, small shop-keepers, and lodging-house keepers, in which capacities they often find kind assistance from *ci-devant* male acquaintances, who are only too glad to second their endeavours. Others, again, devote their energies and their savings to preying in their turn, as keepers or *attachées* of brothels and other disorderly establishments, upon the class of male and female victims they themselves have emerged from.

The most prudish will doubtless agree with me, that an important fraction of ex-prostitutes may be accounted for in the last of these categories. Such, indeed – as reformatories of the kind hitherto opened have been notoriously restricted in their operation – has been the customary theoretical disposition of all, or almost all, who were supposed not to die in the ranks or of supervening illnesses. On reflection, too, the reader may, perhaps, acquiesce in some occasional re-entrances into society through the portals of labour. Emigration also, under its present easy conditions, may be admitted to be an outlet to a certain extent.

When, however, I suggest an enormous and continual action of wedlock upon prostitution, I am quite prepared for the smile of incredulity and the frown of censure from many whose notions of caste, propriety, and so forth, preclude their entertaining for a moment a proposition which would to them appear fraught with scandal, and because scandalous, preposterous. But let me tell the sceptic that this is a matter which, though heretofore it has attracted the attention of a few, will hereafter speak to society as with the voice of a trumpet. . . . The ball is rolling, the Rubicon has been crossed by many who have not been drowned in the attempt, nor found a state of things on the other side more distasteful than compulsory celibacy; and I apprehend that if some of our social marriage enactments are not repealed by acclamation or tacitly, I shall live to see a very large increase in concubinage and the marriages of prostitutes.

There are thousands of fathers, and what is worse, mothers of families, in every rank and occupation of life, who have done much evil, I fear, by the attempt to set up the worship of society in association with that of Mammon. Wholesale dealers in so-called respectability, but screwing out scanty halfpenny-worths of brotherly love, they have passed a marriage code in the joint names of these false divinities, which renders day by day more difficult the union of youth and love unsanctified by money and position. As this goes on, we see more and more of our maidens pining on the stem of single blessedness, more and more of our young men resigning themselves first, for a time, to miscellaneous fornication, then to systematic concubinage, and, of course for all this, none the richer or more eligible in the eyes of society, at last to a *mésalliance*.

I need not enlarge upon the social offence of one who thus practically lessens the number of prostitutes. All reflective men must appreciate in common the sad distress and shame which may accrue to his family, the depravity of his taste, who could consider it a triumph to bear off a battered prize from other competitors, and his insanity, who should dream of avoiding detection, or indulge the hope that, after detection, his false step could be forgotten or forgiven by the world. All can compassionate the temporary weakness of a mind which could esteem the permanent possession of a tainted woman worth the sacrifice of home and social ties. All are at liberty to predict his future sadness, if not misery; though we are apt to err in supposing that the woman purchased at this sacrifice has no affection to return to him, no gratitude, no feeling, no good taste. And, I confess, I have occasionally joined the very worldly and immoral cry against the folly of a man who contrives to make an indissoluble bond of a silken thread which he might have rent at his own will and pleasure – who pays so dearly for the ownership of that which, by a little management, he might have occupied from year to year at will, for next to nothing. These are all everyday platitudes, and unfortunately in such common request that men may gather them at the street corners.

* * *

There are persons who deem the Haymarket and the Argyll Rooms – because, I presume, being adjacent to the Opera House, these places come betwixt the wind and their fine susceptibilities – at once the Alpha and the Omega of prostitution, and would exterminate the vice and its practitioners at one fell swoop, by a bonfire, in the Regent Circus. These will clamour, that the evil is over-magnified when each harlot is called a harlot, because this enlargement of the field of operations puts an end to all nonsensical proposals of high-handed suppression. I use none but their own weapons, when I marshal in the ranks of prostitution each woman who, in a pure society, would properly be so construed. But the accumulation to be dealt with thus becomes so frightful, that all who can read and think will agree with me, that management and regulation of 'the greatest social evil' by the baton or the pillory, grateful though it might be to Exeter Hall,[32] would be neither effective nor perhaps politic.

The hand of an Englishman should be as withered before it advocated the forcible suppression of this vice, as must be the foolish brain that could plot it. Virtue and vice, as we all know, are no subjects for enactment. To protest against the latter's concentration is as futile and absurd as to argue against the herding of nobles or *parvenus*, tradesmen or manufacturers, criminals or paupers. Secrecy would be more fraught than publicity with danger to individuals and the public; diffusion would be lunacy on grounds both of morals and policy. The existing regulations are adequate for public protection and order, which are all the judicious can at present hope for; anything further in that direction we are certainly not prepared for. The Home Secretary who should attempt anything like coercion would soon have his hands full indeed. We are already *policés* [organized] enough – we are already on the verge of excess. . . .

I repeat that prostitution is a transitory state, through which an untold number of British women are ever on their passage. Until preventive measures . . . shall have been considerately adopted – and thereafter, too, if needful, for I am no nostrum-monger – it is the duty, and it should be the business of us all, in the interest of the commonwealth, to see these women through that state, so as to save harmless as much as may be of the bodies and souls of them. And the commonwealth's interest in it is this – that there is never a one among all of these whose partners in vice may not sometime become

75

the husbands of other women, and fathers of English children; never a one of them but may herself, when the shadow is past, become the wife of an Englishman and the mother of his offspring; that multitudes are mothers before they become prostitutes, and other multitudes become mothers during their evil career. If the race of the people is of no concern to the State, then has the State no interest in arresting its vitiation. But if this concern and this interest be admitted, then arises the necessity for depriving prostitution not only of its moral, but of its physical venom also. . . .

3

DISEASES THE RESULT OF
PROSTITUTION

I HAVE now to consider one or two of the most ordinary consequences of promiscuous intercourse. In passing through (as she
generally does, whether rising or falling in the scale) this phase of
her career, the prostitute almost inevitably contracts some form of
the contagious . . . diseases, which in medicine we term 'venereal'.
How these are passed from sex to sex and back again, *ad infinitum*,
it were superfluous here to illustrate. I have treated at length elsewhere, under the head of specific disease, of the laws which govern
these complaints, and of the influences which favour their diffusion,
and the reader will, I dare say, gladly dispense with the introduction
of those topics here. I propose, however, in the following pages, to
offer some idea of their importance, as being the first and foremost of
the effects of prostitution coming under the notice of the surgeon.

★   ★   ★

Until I pointed out the data, some twelve years ago, neither the profession nor the public recognized the fact that one-half the out-
patients at our leading public hospitals came there in consequence
of being affected with venereal diseases. The . . . statistical tables
which I published are now admitted to have brought about the
change in legislation which I shall have hereafter to chronicle. . . .

It would appear . . . that two-thirds of the male applicants for
relief at [the Royal Free Hospital] have recourse to it on account of
venereal affections; and it would seem probable that this has been
going on for twenty-six years at the least. . . .

Surgeons to the Royal Free . . . agree that the proportion of
venereal diseases is very large, and that even the physicians see
among their cases a large proportion of syphilitic complaints, affecting not only the external but the internal parts of the body. . . .

I am disposed to attribute some share in the diminished virulence of venereal complaints to the opening of this and other perfectly free institutions, together with a slight increase of cleanliness among the poor – though by no means proportional, as yet, to the increase of water supply – the institution of public baths, and the greater cheapness of soap and clothing. . . .

It appears . . . from [the] statistics that about one in three soldiers suffers from some venereal complaint. . . . In the French Army . . . at present only 97 per 1,000 men come into hospital for these venereal affections, showing that these complaints are $2\frac{1}{2}$ times more common in England than in France, not one in ten suffering abroad, instead of one in three as in England. . . . Let us hope that the measures I recommended twelve years ago, and now on the point of being carried out in our garrison towns, may render the English soldier as free from such complaints as his Continental confrères.

* * *

I understand that a mild mercurial treatment is usually pursued in the army, for hard sores especially. Some surgeons give no mercury; but this depends upon the discretion of the individual. . . .

It is cheering . . . to observe that the absolute deaths in the last decennial period upon an aggregate of 254,597 men numbered only 17; and happily, also, we now rarely meet with those losses of the palate, nose, or portions of the cranium which our museums show must formerly have been frequent. . . .

[In 1865, in the navy], 4,313 cases of syphilis were under treatment, of which 130 were invalided. . . . Venereal diseases . . . are more common among soldiers than among sailors, owing, probably, to the more limited opportunities of becoming infected which the profession of the latter exposes them to. . . .

In the merchant service, one in every three patients who applies to the hospital suffers from venereal disease. . . .

As far, then, as we may judge . . . venereal diseases are still very common among large bodies of otherwise healthy males engaged in the public service. At the same time, scurvy and hospital gangrene have nearly disappeared from the reports. The returns do not enable us to arrive at any accurate conclusion how far they incapacitate their victims from duty. Dr Wilson,[33] who must be supposed to be a competent judge, inasmuch as he has compiled the returns, told me in 1857 that on an average each man so affected [was] incapacitated from doing duty for a month. In the army, his stay in hospital has been averaged at six weeks. In the return furnished by Mr Busk,[34] the average stay in hospital is stated to be twenty-two days; this is similar to that in the army; and during five years the expense of venereal patients was £4,165.

I doubt whether venereal complaints, although evidently more severe formerly, were ever more common than at present, or whether, since syphilis was first treated in hospitals, the large proportion . . . (namely two out of three out-patients at the Free Hospital, nearly one in two at St Bartholomew's, one out of every three at the *Dreadnought*, one out of four in the army, one out of seven in the navy) at any former period suffered from venereal disease. And yet many believe that the disease is declining. That such is not the case, if number be any criterion, must be admitted by all who weigh well the statistics, and compare them with the statements met with in nearly all the books that have treated of syphilis. . . .

If my inferences are correct, that venereal diseases, though decreasing in virulence, are numerically as prevalent as ever, where single men are massed together, is it not time to consider, whether in the present advanced state of civilization, some methodical steps should not be taken still further to mitigate and, as nearly as may be, eradicate the evil, more especially as we have so successfully operated against many others of 'the thousand natural shocks that flesh is heir to'?

Truth demands the acknowledgment that the individual affections both in England and on the Continent, are less severe in the present day. In but few cases do the symptoms run high, or is the patient permanently crippled by the disease. I myself can testify to enormous changes in this respect during the last twenty years. The frightful cases, attended with the loss of the nose, palate, etc., which formerly were really not uncommon, are now very rare either in hospitals or in private practice. The weekly average of deaths from syphilis in London, within the last ten years, varies from 1·6 to 4·3. Phagedaena, or 'the black lion of Portugal', was formerly to be met with weekly in our hospitals. It is now an exceptional case. Sir Astley Cooper[35] states, that in the St Giles's Workhouse at one time and in one room there were seven of these terrible cases, of which five were fatal. I need not say that, thanks to the improved treatment, and the many channels of relief available to the poor, these wholesale

79

calamities are put a stop to, although an isolated case . . . may every now and then result in a fatal termination. . . .

I cannot pretend to offer an opinion as to the general increase or decrease of these complaints in private practice. There is in our profession very little interchange of notes and statistics, and no organized correspondence with any body or society, and I fancy no medical man could draw a sound deduction as to the greater or less prevalence of any particular disease from the state of his own practice. He who should believe and say disease was extravagantly rife in London because he individually happened to be much in vogue, would deliver himself of as notable a fallacy, I apprehend, as another who should declare it was totally extinct, because from being out of repute, out of date, out of the stream, or for some other of the thousand reasons which sway the British public, he never happened to see a patient at all.

Each one, however, may without difficulty contribute a little information to the common stock by analysing the mass of cases which are presented to him. I shall give here one or two opinions, resulting from my own experience, which may, perhaps, be hereafter of value to others. . . .

In the first place – the venereal affections now seen in private practice are slight. Patients come to the medical man early. The *mauvaise honte*, which formerly acted to their prejudice, is passing away, and the necessity for immediate treatment generally admitted. To this cause I attribute to a great extent the mildness of the disease, and the rapidity of cure in the majority of cases. No doubt can exist that improved treatment and a more correct diagnosis are operating in the same direction; science has been assisted by the almost complete abstinence of the upper classes generally from intoxication, though not from liquor, and the liberal ablutions now so much and so beneficially in fashion.

The loss of the virile organ is, nowadays, a thing almost unheard of in private practice. A surgeon might practise in London for many years without gaining any experience of the affection of the bones of the nose which causes that organ to fall in. It is true that we occasionally meet with an obstinate case of this affection in highly strumous patients, but even these, under appropriate treatment, escape the sad deformity, and ultimately recover. I have, every now and then, cases of tertiary symptoms, which return again and again, and offer most rebellious instances of the virulence of the disease amongst the weak and debilitated; but still death from syphilis is almost unheard of in private practice. I did see one some time ago. It came on gradually from a want of rallying power in the system, and a few tubercles were found in the lungs. It is to be regretted that in the present day the indurated sore is not more rare, attended as it is with many sad sequelae. Secondary symptoms are not severe, but, although slight, they linger on for months, now better, now worse, until the powers of the system, if well supported, get the better of the affections of the tongue or the eruption on the skin. Rarely, now, are the deeper structures affected, and patients generally, if not very injudiciously treated, completely recover within a reasonable time.

The results of private practice bear out the statistics from the public institutions, that gonorrhoea is the most frequent of the venereal affections. It no longer, however, takes the formidable shapes of bygone times, although it is often to the full as tiresome from assuming the chronic form.

I am often obliged to remind nervous patients who complain of tardy cures, that though they have to thank advancing science for such mild results as now form the penalty of their frailty, they must not expect a day when the complaint is to be divested of all pain or annoyance. Neither the disease nor our treatment are in general so much to be blamed for the worst phases which the former even now occasionally assumes, as the naturally bad constitution of the sufferer or the perverse industry he has applied to the debilitation of a sound one. He has oftentimes his own neglect to thank for doubled and trebled suffering – often his own folly in bringing to us only the reversion of a case complicated, and perhaps aggravated, by one or other of the villainous quacksalvers who are still permitted to flaunt their nostrums in the public face, to gull, to swindle, and to kill.

The observations I made in 1857 on the extortion of quacks [apply] equally to the subject in 1869, and I allow the case which appeared in my last edition to remain as a beacon to warn the unwary. A gentleman who believed himself to be suffering from spermatorrhoea[36] went to a noted quack and paid his usual fee. A specimen of his urine was immediately demanded, and on examination under a microscope, pronounced to be full of spermatozoa. The patient showed unmistakable signs of alarm, and the quack, finding he had the proper sort of customer, boldly predicted speedy death, to be averted only by the purchase of a cure for fifty pounds. The first call of nine pounds on account of this sum was paid on the spot, and the remainder within a few days. The patient was then, I am assured, presented with a large box of medicines, ready packed, and desired to keep in a room at the same temperature for twenty-eight weeks, or thereabouts, and not attempt to breathe the outer air. After some weeks of unrewarded perseverance in this régime, the unhappy patient again sought the presence of the wizard, and complained that he felt no better. He was asked, 'How could he expect it? Had he not disobeyed? His presence there was proof enough of that!' He pleaded in vain, that to keep his room for twenty-eight weeks, if not impossible, would be his ruin, and was told that, having by his own act removed the responsibility from the learned doctor's shoulders, their contract was at an end, and he must now put up with the possible ill consequences, and the certain loss of his money. It was under these circumstances that he came to me, in a highly nervous state, and of course much annoyed at being bereft of fifty pounds by this 'microscope dodge'. In three weeks he recovered, and would not have rushed, as he did, into the courts of law but for the impudent plea set up for not returning the money after failure of the consideration. The recipient of the fifty pounds actually stated that the deluded one had been guilty of masturbation, and therefore could not show his face in court. The challenge was accepted, and the infamous imputation of course faded away. I cannot show the sequel better than by quoting the following passage from the judgment of the court:

I have not the slightest doubt upon this case – that it is a case for damages, and that the plaintiff is entitled to recover the whole of the sum claimed. I think it is highly creditable to the plaintiff that he had the moral courage to come into court and expose this transaction; and as to the agency, the assistant, whoever he may be, has certainly committed a gross fraud, and one cannot help feeling warmly that this fraud was practised. At the same time one cannot help seeing as to ——— —— not having been present at the interviews, that this is a mere stratagem to secure himself against the consequences of being brought into a court of justice; and the whole of the case, I think, is very discreditable to the defendant, and the plaintiff is entitled to the judgment of the court for the whole of the amount sued for. One cannot help saying that the whole case is most discreditable and disgusting, and I shall allow the highest expenses to the witnesses.

The editor of the *Lancet* observed, in conclusion of his remarks upon this case:

How long is this system to continue? It is a disgrace to the laws, which falsely pretend to regulate practitioners of medicine and to protect the public, that such things are allowed. The case in question is simply an illustration of a system so ruinous, so devastating, so fatal to its victims, that it calls loudly for legislative interference. Laws, however framed, will probably be inadequate altogether to suppress these outrages upon humanity; but legislation may do something to mitigate and arrest them. If we are to have laws for the protection of women, and the suppression of obscene publications, why should we not have an Act of Parliament to suppress a traffic which in its consequences is equally detrimental to the health and happiness of a large portion of the public?*

* [*Lancet*, 1857, II. 146.]

4

EXISTING PROVISION FOR THE CONTROL AND RELIEF OF PROSTITUTES

I HAVE now passed in review before the reader the leading features of prostitution, as exhibited in this country, and I have shown him the vast extent of the evil, by placing before him the numbers of the women who snatch a precarious living from this life of sin. Some, as we have seen, enjoy in their turn, for a brief season, a pre-eminence in guilt, on whom large sums are lavished, to be recklessly squandered on the adornment of their bodies, and indulgence in sensual excesses, without thought for the time of want and misery that surely overtakes the prostitute who prolongs the pursuit of her calling beyond her prime to that sad period when health, and youth, and beauty, and all that renders woman attractive, are no longer hers; while others, and these the vast majority, are forced to give, in exchange for the bare means of keeping life, all that makes life worth having, and are oft-times sunk so low as to abandon their bodies for the poor return of a few paltry pence. The ruin wrought on these wretched women is bad enough, but, as we have seen, it is not all, or nearly all, the evil produced by the system. Vice does not hide itself, it throngs our streets, intrudes into our parks and theatres, and other places of resort, bringing to the foolish temptation, and knowledge of sin to the innocent; it invades the very sanctuary of home, destroying conjugal happiness, and blighting the hopes of parents.

Nor is it indirectly only that society is injured; we have seen that prostitutes do not, as is generally supposed, die in harness; but that, on the contrary, they for the most part become, sooner or later, with tarnished bodies and polluted minds, wives and mothers; while among some classes of the people the moral sentiment is so depraved, that the woman who lives by the hire of her person is received on almost equal terms to social intercourse. It is clear, then, that though we may call these women outcasts and pariahs, they have a powerful influence for evil on all ranks of the community. The moral injury inflicted on society by prostitution is incalculable; the physical injury is at least as great.

Let us take the case of London: in this city, as the return shows, there are 6,515 women known to the police to be prostitutes; it is not too much to say that out of every four of these women one at least is diseased, so that we have among us more than 1,500, at a moderate computation, human beings daily engaged in the occupation of spreading abroad a loathsome poison, the effects of which are not even confined to the partakers of their sin, but are too often transmitted to his issue, and bear their fruits in tottering limbs and tainted blood. Broken constitutions, sickly bodies, and feeble minds are times out of number the work of the prostitute. In a few words, then, prostitution consigns to a life of degradation thousands of our female population, ruining them utterly body and soul, who in their turn retaliate on society the wrong inflicted on themselves. It makes our streets unfit thoroughfares for the modest, and a reproach to us when compared with the decency observable in foreign cities. It exercises an evil influence on the nation at large, depraving the minds and lowering the moral tone. It is the cause of disease, premature decay, untimely death. Having thus become to a certain extent acquainted with the evil whose ravages we desire to mitigate, we may now shortly examine the actual state of the law with regard to it – that is, what pressure it is in the power of the authorities to exercise upon it, and how far that power is exerted.

★ ★ ★

The attitude assumed by the law towards prostitution may be briefly stated as follows:

It requires the police to repress flagrant acts of indecency and disorder in the streets and places of public resort;

It restrains the opening of theatres and places of amusement or refreshment without a licence, which must be applied for annually, and is continued only during good behaviour, thereby making it the interest of managers and proprietors to discountenance gross disorders, and to maintain so far as possible the outward forms of decorum in their establishments;

It prohibits the opening of refreshment houses during certain hours of the night, a prohibition imposed, notwithstanding the hardship thereby inflicted on some classes of workmen, for the purpose of putting an end, if possible, to the shameless debauchery nightly exhibited in the Haymarket and its environs;

It encourages the prosecution of keepers of brothels and other disorderly houses;

But it ignores the existence of prostitution as a system, exerting its authority in those cases only which, by open contempt for order and decency, obtrude into notice and demand repression. Men and women are, in fact, left in this matter to their own consciences; and so long as they respect public decency, their private conduct passes unchallenged, while the different parishes are left to decide for themselves whether or not they will permit known prostitutes to find shelter within their borders. How far this state of the law is wise and right will form the subject of consideration in a future chapter. One result of prostitution, with the evil and extent of which we dealt in the preceding chapter, has forced into action on behalf of certain classes and certain districts an unwilling legislature; the result of that action we shall presently consider, but first of all we will glance at the means at present provided for alleviating disease.

LOCK HOSPITAL

If we turn to London, a city of 3,000,000 souls, we find but ONE institution *specially* devoted to the treatment of venereal diseases – the LOCK HOSPITAL, formerly of Southwark, afterwards of Grosvenor Place, now of Westbourne Green and Dean Street, Soho, the existence of which for more than a century was one continued struggle. Formerly, both male and female patients were received at Westbourne Green; now females only are taken in there, the male patients having been transferred to the branch establishment in Dean Street, Soho, which contains 30 beds, though the funds of the institution only admit of 15 being occupied at present. Out-patients, both male and female, are attended to at Dean Street, and apply in large numbers. In 1868, 5,052 males and 800 females were treated there as out-patients. In connexion with the Female Hospital at Westbourne, is the Asylum, containing an average of about 60 inmates, but capable of receiving 80, for the reformation of patients who have been cured in the hospital.

A new wing, called the Prince of Wales's Wing, has been recently added to the female division of this hospital. The cost of the erection for building alone was £9,800, and when swelled by the sums expended on foundations, gas stoves, baths, fittings, furniture, and everything required for habitation, amounted to £12,000. It contains 75 beds, which would make the cost £160 per bed. But this would be an unfair estimate, because the new part contains all the kitchens, store-rooms, and other offices required for 150 patients, together with all the residents' rooms. The parts of the old building previously devoted to these purposes have now been either converted into wards, or given up to the use of the asylum. In 1867, 169 ordinary patients were admitted, with an average stay in hospital of 50 days each. The daily average, therefore, of ordinary patients present throughout the year was 23·15. . . .

GUY'S HOSPITAL

. . . Out of 700 beds the hospital devotes 28 to male venereal cases, and 30 to female. During the year 1868, there were treated in the hospital 422 cases of syphilis. Of these 123 males and 124 females were cured; 69 males were relieved and 87 females; 8 males left unrelieved, and 5 females; 1 male died, and 1 female, and the cause of the deaths was sloughing of the vulva, and laryingeal disease.

★　★　★

The proportion of venereal out-patients seen at this hospital are about 43 per cent.

★　★　★

ST BARTHOLOMEW'S HOSPITAL

Having been educated at this hospital, I may be pardoned for rejoicing at the noble prominence my *Alma Mater* has been enabled to assume in alleviating the miseries of humanity. This present work of mine may probably be traceable to the unequalled opportunities this noble institution afforded me of seeing venereal affections in the commencement of my studies, and it still continues to devote more wards to the treatment of venereal cases than does any other general hospital.

I have already stated . . . that this institution contains 75 beds, given up to venereal cases. There are 25 devoted to males and 50 to females, 597 cases were treated in the hospital for syphilis and other specific complaints in the year 1868, and, as we have seen, . . . more than half the out-patients are sufferers from venereal affections.

* * *

I regret to say that the indecent system of exposing females before the whole class of students is still pursued, and that the employment of the speculum is the exception, not the rule. It is with regret I mention the shortcomings of my *Alma Mater*. Before another edition of this book appears, I trust I may be able to chronicle that every woman entering the venereal wards is examined with the speculum; that the examinations are made in a separate ward or behind a screen raised at the farther extremity, and thus separated from the gaze of her fellow-sufferers; and that only a few pupils are allowed to be present at a time.

* * *

CONTAGIOUS DISEASES ACT

However much it may be the duty of the State to leave for settlement to the individual conscience all questions of morals and religion, it can hardly be seriously contended that it is right to abandon to the care of the improvident and profligate the restraining of contagious maladies, yet this, except in a few military and naval stations, is virtually the case in England. A woman who knows herself to be diseased, is free to invite all comers to the enjoyment of her person, and to spread among them deadly contagion. The total of venereal beds is, as we have seen, in St Bartholomew's, 75; in Guy's, 58; in Middlesex, 20; in the Royal Free, 26; in the Lock, exclusive of those required by Government, 30. Thus, although the population of London numbers over 3,000,000, there are only 155 beds given up to females labouring under venereal affections, if we deduct the 120 beds at the Lock Hospital devoted to the Government patients sent there from Woolwich, Aldershot, and other garrison towns.

These figures speak for themselves, and when we remember the deadly character of the disease with which we have to contend, the strong temptations that lead to its contraction, and the vast numbers who yield to that temptation, and compare them with the means at our disposal for supplying an antidote to the poison, we may well marvel at the indifference of society and the supineness of Government. But if we can ill excuse the laws, which afford no protection to those who, after all, are comparatively free agents, what shall we say of them, if we find them placing thousands of men every year in the utmost jeopardy, compelling them almost, for the convenience of the State, to have recourse to the prostitution by which they are surrounded, and yet providing for them no means of safety or adequate relief? It is hardly credible that, until a few years ago, this was the case in England. At length in 1864 the injury inflicted by this apathy on our soldiers and sailors, and the loss sustained by the public purse, seem to have touched the conscience or the cupidity of the legislature, and in that year an Act was passed, ... having for its object the remedy of the evils to which the army and navy are exposed; its provisions, however, proved totally inadequate to meet the requirements of the case, and it was followed in 1866 by a more comprehensive measure, ... commonly called the Contagious Diseases Act.

This Act now extends its operation to Canterbury, Dover, Gravesend, Maidstone, Southampton, Winchester, Portsmouth, Plymouth and Devonport, Woolwich, Chatham, Sheerness, Aldershot, Windsor, Colchester, Shorncliffe, the Curragh, Cork, and Queenstown. By the 15th and 16th sections, a justice of the peace, on information being laid before him that a woman, living in any place to which the Act extends, is a common prostitute, and on oath before him substantiating such information, may, if he thinks fit, order that the woman be subject to a periodical medical examination by the visiting surgeon appointed under the provisions of the Act, for any period not exceeding one year, for the purpose of ascertaining at each such examination whether she is affected with a contagious disease; and thereupon she shall be subject to such a periodical medical examination, and the order shall be a sufficient warrant for the visiting surgeon to conduct such examination accordingly. And by the 17th section any woman, in any place to which the Act applies, may, by a submission signed by her, in the presence of, and attested by the superintendent of police, subject herself to a periodical examination under this Act for any period not exceeding one year. Any woman found on examination to be diseased, may either go herself, or will be apprehended and sent, to some hospital certified for the reception and detention of Government patients. The reception of a woman in a certified hospital by the managers or persons having the management or control thereof shall be deemed to be an undertaking by them to provide for her care, treatment, lodging, clothing and food during her detention in hospital. This period of detention is limited to three months, or, on the certificate prescribed by the Act that further detention is necessary, to a further period of six months, making nine months in the whole. If a woman considers herself detained in hospital too long, she may apply to a justice for an order of discharge.

Prostitutes refusing to conform to the provisions of this Act are liable to be punished by imprisonment, and anyone permitting a woman who to his knowledge is suffering from a contagious disease, to use his house for the purpose of prostitution shall, in addition to the other consequences to which he may be liable for keeping a disorderly house, be liable to six months imprisonment with or without hard labour. The appointment of the necessary surgeons, inspectors of hospitals, and other officers, is intrusted to the Admiralty and War Offices, by whom also hospitals may be provided and certified for use, and all expenses incurred in the execution of the Act must be defrayed. The carrying out of the Act in the minor details is of course intrusted to the police.

It is also provided that adequate provision must be made by the several hospitals for the moral and religious instruction of the women detained in them under this Act. We have already seen that a considerable number of beds have been secured at the Lock Hospital for the use of Government patients. The most admirable arrangements have been adopted at this institution for the examination and treatment of the patients committed to its care, and as the possibility of carrying out an act having for its object the diminution of disease forms an important element in considering the advisability of further extending its sphere of usefulness, I shall offer no apology for relating pretty fully the method pursued in this institution.

LOCK HOSPITAL

I was anxious to see the working of the existing Government Lock Hospital, and Mr J. Lane[37] kindly allowed me to accompany him, and explained everything on my visit in October, 1868.

The patients (female) are lodged in a new wing; the wards are lofty, and kept scrupulously clean. Each inmate has a separate bed, provided with three blankets, and a hair mattress, an extra blanket being given in winter. Each patient has two pannikins, a half-pint and a pint tin can, with a pewter spoon and a steel knife and fork; and a little box in which she may keep her things is placed near her bed. The patients are not allowed to go into other wards, but there is an open court in which they take exercise, and they have a sort of hospital dress in place of their own clothes, which are left under the care of the matron. At the head of the bed hangs a towel.

In a little room at the end of the ward water is laid on, and copper basins are hung by a chain to the wall; these basins are kept for the women to wash their faces. This arrangement is specially made to prevent any possible contagion. Fixed to the floor is a bidet, across which the female sits. There is here an admirable device for facilitating the cleansing of the private parts; by... means [of] a brass syringe, with a long pewter ball, and holding, say six ounces, she injects the lotion, and the waste fluid runs away on opening a plug fixed in the bottom of the bidet. The only improvement I could suggest was that each patient be furnished with two small napkins to dry the organs after injection. The patient always uses an injection before presenting herself to the surgeon, in order that the organs may be in a proper condition for examination, and I must say the cleanliness shown does great credit to the nurses who manage the wards.

The inspections are conducted in the following manner. The women are introduced one at a time from the wards by one nurse into a special room, containing a properly-raised bed, with feet, similar to the one in use on the Continent. The patient ascends the steps placed by the side of the bed, lays down, places her feet in the slippers arranged for the purpose, and the house surgeon separates the labia to see if there are any sores. If no suspicion of these exists, and if the female is suffering from discharge, the speculum is at once employed. In this institution several sizes are used, and they are silvered and covered with india-rubber. The head nurse after each examination washes the speculum in a solution of permanganate of potash, then wipes it carefully, oils it ready for the next examination, so that the surgeon loses no time, and the examinations are conducted with great rapidity. In the course of one hour and three-quarters I assisted in the thorough examination of 58 women with the speculum.

In this institution the house surgeon examines the women; the surgeon superintending and prescribing the remedies.

Mr J. Lane, in a recent paper, has so well described the method of treatment adopted by him, that I shall give an account of it in his own words:

Since the admission of patients into this hospital, under the Contagious Diseases Act, from Woolwich and other military districts, the treatment of uterine and vaginal discharges has constituted a large part of its practice. In fact, in 1867, as many as 58 per cent, and in 1868, 65 per cent of the class of patients alluded to, were placed under treatment for this form of disease alone, uncomplicated by any symptom of a syphilitic character, either primary or secondary. These patients are, for the most part, strong, healthy girls, aged from 17 to 25, well fed, and in good condition. Their disease appears to be entirely local, both in its origin and character. It arises, as I believe, in the great majority of cases, simply from the continual irritation and excitement of the generative organs consequent upon their mode of life, though it may be caused, no doubt, occasionally by direct contagion from urethral discharges in the male. The secretion, when they first come under observation, is of an obviously purulent or muco-purulent character, and evidence of its contagiousness is afforded by the fact (as I am informed) that nearly all of them have been accused of communicating disease before being subjected to examination. It is remarkable how little pain or inconvenience is suffered by these patients; usually they make no complaint whatever, and many of them are unaware that anything whatever is the matter with them, although, when examined with the speculum, a profuse discharge, derived chiefly from the uterus, is found lodged in the upper part of the vagina. Associated with this, especially in the more chronic cases, abrasions of the epithelium excoriations, or superficial ulcerations on the vaginal portion of the cervix uteri are very frequently seen. Anything approaching to an inflammatory condition, to which the terms acute gonorrhoea or vaginitis might be applied, is uncommon, and when met with, it is usually in young girls, as yet unseasoned to a life of prostitution. Incidental complications, of a painful character, such as labial abscess, or inflammatory bubo, are occasionally seen, but are not of frequent occurrence.

An external examination alone is quite insufficient for the discovery of these complaints. Purulent secretions from the vulva or lower part of the vagina are, of course, evident enough; but a profuse uterine discharge may be present, and no trace of it be visible until the speculum is employed. There is, however, a considerable difference in women in this respect; in some, the vagina appears to be equally contractile throughout its whole length, and therefore, any secretion formed in it, or entering it, speedily appears externally; while in others, and these are the majority, its contractility is much less at the upper than at the lower part, and discharges are consequently retained in the former situation.

When these discharges are of purely local origin, and there is no constitutional fault, their cure may be speedily effected by local applications. The plan commonly pursued at the Lock Hospital is to make the patients use vaginal injections for themselves three or four times daily. The lotions employed are the diluted liquor plumbi subacetatis, or solutions of sulphate of zinc, alum, or tannin, in the proportion of five grains to the ounce of water. The syringes are large enough to hold six ounces of the lotion, and have a pipe long enough to reach the upper part of the vagina readily. Both these points are important, for the syringes commonly used will not contain sufficient fluid to wash out the canal effectually, and the pipe affixed to them will not admit of its reaching the upper part of the vagina at all. When the vaginal mucous membrane is inflamed and tender, the house surgeon, when the speculum is used, which is at least twice a week in all these cases, inserts a strip of lint dipped in the lead-lotion, and this is allowed to remain for three or four hours. If the inflammation be acute, the application of the strip of lint is repeated daily through a small speculum. By these means, discharges proceeding from the vagina may usually be cured in a few days, but the injections should be continued as long as any abnormal uterine secretions are observed, for the latter, if not frequently washed away, will be likely to re-excite disease in the vaginal mucous membrane.*

* * *

The medical officers told me, in reply to my inquiries, that there had been occasional disturbances among the patients. The nurse first

* [James R. Lane, 'Notes on the Practice of the London Female Lock Hospital', *British Medical Journal*, 1868, II. 592.]

tries to stop any outbreak of temper; if unsuccessful, the house surgeon is appealed to, and if he fails, the girl is conveyed to the police
station by the hospital porter, who is empowered to act as a police
constable in relation to these patients, who are then liable to two
months' imprisonment.

I have little to say about the patients; in appearance they are not
generally prepossessing; a few among those whom I saw were young,
and looked middle-aged and plain. The primary syphilitic affections
were few, but the diseases of the uterus numerous, similar to those I
witness in private practice. . . .

The following is the scale of dietary at the hospital:

ORDINARY

Breakfast	...	...	8 oz. Bread; ½ pint Cocoa.
Dinner	...	...	Five days – ½ lb. Meat; ½ lb. Potatoes.
			Two days – 1 pint Soup; Soup Meat.
			1½ oz. Rice.
Tea ...	...	...	6 oz. Bread; ½ pint Tea.
Supper	...	...	1 pint Gruel.

MEAT DIET

Breakfast	...	...	As above.
Dinner	...	...	½ lb. Meat; ½ lb. Potatoes, every day.
Tea ...	...	...	6 oz. Bread; ½ pint Tea.
Supper	...	...	1 pint Gruel.

BEEF TEA AND PUDDING DIET

Breakfast	...	...	As above, and 1 pint of Milk.
Dinner	...	...	1 pint Beef Tea; 2 oz. Rice in a pudding.
Tea ...	...	...	As above.
Supper	...	...	1 pint Gruel.

Mutton Chop or Fish, when ordered, instead of Meat Diet or ordinary.
Rice occasionally instead of Potatoes.
Extras : Porter, Wine, Spirits and Milk.

ALDERSHOT HOSPITAL

The Aldershot hospital is situate a short distance from the camp on a
rising ground, and consists of a series of one-storied huts, made of
galvanized iron. The day of my visit was a very cold one, but I found
the interior warm and comfortable. It contains six wards, arranged

for the accommodation of 90 patients. Three of these wards are fitted up with 14 beds each; two with 20; the other, a smaller one, with eight only – giving 90 beds in all. Each patient has a folding bed to herself, which is kept scrupulously clean, and done up as a hammock during the day, the patients having to take their meals and pass the day in the wards.

★ ★ ★

So admirable are the arrangements at this institution, that one thing only came under my notice that could possibly operate as a drawback to the health and comfort of the inmates. The view from the windows, which are kept constantly closed, is interrupted by means of blinds and whitened glass, and a certain amount of light and air thereby excluded. This is to be regretted, but seems absolutely necessary, as, in consequence of the close proximity of the hospital to a much frequented road, great difficulty was experienced previously to the adoption of this course, in keeping the inmates from presenting themselves at the windows, and holding conversations with soldiers and others outside the building. . . .

Every patient received into the hospital is required to take a bath immediately on her admittance; her clothes also are taken from her, and well fumigated and washed; they are then made up into neat packages, and are not returned until her time for leaving the hospital has arrived. For her use in the meantime a good supply of warm clothing is provided by the Government. The patients in each ward that I inspected seemed to be in good health, and were comely looking girls, appearing to great advantage in the hospital uniform. The demeanour of these women, as we passed along, was most respectful; there was no noise, no bad language, no sullenness, no levity. The patients are employed when convalescent in laundry and kitchen work, under the superintendence of a paid laundress and cook. In addition to this they make their own clothes, and keep them in proper repair. At the time of my visit they were engaged in making 40 sets of clothing for the use of the Lock Hospital then about to be opened at Cork. Many of the women, on admission, are found totally ignorant of ordinary domestic duties; but great pains in this respect are taken with them during the period of their detention, so that on leaving they are generally found to have become decent needle- and washerwomen, and to have acquired sufficient knowledge of cooking to enable them to dress plain joints and vegetables. The good done by this means has been shown in more than one instance, where a woman so benefited by instruction, has taken service, almost directly after receiving her discharge from the hospital. The patients are permitted to take a walk daily in an exercising ground behind the hospital. I understand that perfect order is maintained among the older residents without much interference on the part of the surgeon, who has unbounded authority, though it requires great tact and determination on his part to reduce newcomers to a proper state of submission and obedience. Doubtless, also, the dread of not being cured rapidly, and thus having their stay in hospital prolonged, helps materially in the task of controlling these, at other times, lawless women; they are also overlooked by a superior class of nurse, and the police in uniform are always to be found at the hospital gate, which is closed to the public. When the patient is discharged she is free, if she pleases, to return to her old haunts; but, if she desires it, she can be placed in an asylum, or if she has friends willing to receive her, and to whom she is willing to go, she is sent to them at the expense of the Government. The good effect of the system inaugurated in this country by the Contagious Diseases Act is apparent even in those women who return to their abandoned ways. They no longer come to the periodical inspections in rags and dirt, but present on these occasions quite an altered appearance; some, as I am informed, even staying at home previously to presenting themselves, to wash the little linen they possess, and put their dresses otherwise into a decent state. Thus are these miserable women being humanized little by little, and the Government is doing at Aldershot a very efficient work by very efficient men. . . .

5

PROSTITUTION IN FRANCE

... I PROPOSE ... in this chapter to examine in detail the system adopted in ... France, both as our nearest neighbour, and as the country that has always led the way in the advance of modern civilization and the growth of modern ideas. . . .

The great object of the system adopted in France is to repress private or secret, and to encourage public or avowed prostitution.

I may, however, as well premise by observing that the authorities of Paris by no means pretend to have established a control over the whole prostitution of that city. The *concubinaires* [kept mistresses] they cannot reach. The large sections of superior professional prostitutes, whom the French term *femmes galantes* [gay women] and *lorettes* [women of easy virtue], evade them, as do also vast hordes of the lowest class of strumpets who throng the low quarters and the villages of the Banlieue. . . .

The official registration of common prostitutes . . . is now either on the voluntary demand of the female or by requisition of the *Bureau des Mœurs*. On appearing before this tribunal, the candidate, after declaring her name, age, quality, birth-place, occupation, and domicile, is submitted to a searching examination, as follows. Is she married or single? Has she a father and mother living, and what are their pursuits? Does she reside with them; if not, why not, and when did she leave them? Has she children? How long has she inhabited Paris, and can she be owned there? Has she ever been arrested, and if so, the particulars? Has she previously been a prostitute; if so, the details? Has she had any, and what, education? Has she had any venereal affection? Her motives for the step?

She next proceeds to the *Bureau Sanitaire*, is medically examined, and enrolled in that department. If found diseased, she is consigned to the Saint-Lazare Hospital forthwith. Steps are meanwhile taken to verify her replies at the *Bureau des Mœurs*, and formal communications are now made to the mayor of her native commune, with an appeal for the woman's redemption to her parents. . . .

D

Should the relatives of the girl be willing to receive her, she is remitted to them at the public cost. She, however, frequently refuses to disclose them, or is ignorant of their existence, and it rarely occurs that they reclaim her. If, as has happened, she be a virgin or a minor, she is consigned to a religious establishment. Should spleen or despair cause the step, and she show symptoms of good qualities, immediate attempts are made to change her intention, and she is often sent home, or placed in a reformatory at the public cost. If her parents reside in Paris they are communicated with. All, in fact, that the *Bureau des Mœurs* can do, I should in justice say, I believe to be done, to warn and restrain the female about to enrol herself in the ranks of public prostitution, and only when all has failed is the formality complied with. This formality, which takes the form of a colourable contract or covenant between the prostitute and the authorities, would seem to argue a sort of consciousness on the part of the latter of the entire illegality of the proceedings throughout....

This over, the individual is presumed at liberty to select the category of prostitution in which she will be comprehended. If she is totally destitute, or any arrangement to this effect had been previously entered into, she is registered to a certain licensed house, to whose licensed proprietress she becomes a marked and numbered serf or chattel, to be used or abused, within certain limitations, at discretion. If she has command of capital enough to furnish a lodging of her own, she is provided with a ticket, or *carte*. . . .

On the reverse . . . are printed the following

Obligations and Restrictions imposed on Public Women

Public women, *en carte*, are called upon to present themselves at the dispensary for examination, once at least every fifteen days.

They are called upon to exhibit this card on every request of police officers and agents.

They are forbidden to practise the calling during daylight, or to walk in the thoroughfares until at least half an hour after the public lamps are lighted, or at any season of the year before seven o'clock, or after eleven P.M.

They must be simply and decently clad, so as not to attract attention by the richness, striking colours, or extravagant fashion of their dress.

They must wear some sort of cap or bonnet, and not present themselves bareheaded.

They are strictly forbidden to address men accompanied by females or children, or to address loud or anxious solicitations to any person.

They may not, under any pretext whatever, exhibit themselves at their windows, which must be kept constantly closed and provided with curtains.

They are strictly forbidden to take up a station on the foot-pavement, to form, or walk together, in groups, or to and fro in a narrow space, or to allow themselves to be attended or followed by men.

The neighbourhood of churches and chapels, within a radius of twenty-five yards, the arcades and approaches of the Palais Royal, the Tuileries, the Luxembourg, and the Jardin des Plantes, are interdicted.

The Champs Elysées, the Terrace of the Invalides, the exterior of the Boulevards, the quays, the bridges, and the more unfrequented and obscure localities are alike forbidden.

They are especially forbidden to frequent public establishments or private houses where clandestine prostitution might be facilitated, or to attend *tables-d'hôte*, reside in boarding-houses, or exercise the calling beyond the quarter of the town they reside in.

They are likewise strictly prohibited from sharing lodgings with a kept woman, or other girl, or to reside in furnished lodgings at all without a permit.

Public women must abstain when at home from anything which can give ground for complaints by their neighbours, or the passers-by.

Those who may infringe the above regulations, resist the agents of authority, or give false names or addresses, will incur penalties proportioned to the gravity of the case.

To recapitulate, then: the public women called *filles soumises*, *inscrites*, or *enregistrées*, over whom the *Bureau des Mœurs* of the prefecture of police has cast its net, are divided into two categories:

1. Domiciled in, and registered to certain licensed houses, for whom the keepers of those houses are responsible.

2. Free prostitutes, who are responsible to the authorities direct.

The first, or *filles des maisons*, are known at the Bureaux by their number, and that of the house to which they are *inscrites*, and are termed by themselves *filles à numéro*. Their health is inspected by the official medical staff, at the house of their inscription, once in every week. The second form two sub-classes – viz., women who have their own apartment and furniture, and others who, by special permit, live in furnished lodgings, etc. . . .

[The *Bureau Sanitaire*] was placed upon its present footing in 1828. The medical staff consists of ten superior and ten assistant surgeons. . . .

The inspection, for which the speculum is very frequently used, is performed with all the delicacy consistent with accuracy, and great dispatch; the average time occupied being three minutes, which includes filling up the papers. . . .

The same policy which considers the registration of the prostitute indispensable to public order, dictates the exercise of considerable caution in liberating her from supervision. The formalities which attend . . . the authorized '*radiation*' [striking off the roll] are numerous and strict. The petition must . . . be in writing, and supported by evidence of an intention really and truly to abandon the mode of life. The corroborative demand of an intending husband; of parents or relatives who will be responsible for future conduct; in certain well-authenticated cases, that of one who will secure her as a mistress against future want; or a medical certificate of inability to continue prostitution, all command respect and action, more or less immediate. But the mere profession of changed sentiments is treated with suspicion, and a probation of two or three months under private surveillance is insisted upon. The prayer is granted only on its being made clear that it results from something more than an *intention passagère*, or disgust at the inspection – that means of honest support are more than probably forthcoming, and that public order and salubrity will not be jeopardized by the reappearance of the petitioner as an *insoumise* upon the public streets.

The authorized annual *radiation* during the ten years ending 1854, averaged 258, of whom 24 per annum became wives. The unauthorized averaged 724, and the recaptures 450 per annum, respectively.

The Parisian *maisons de tolérance*, formerly called *bordels*, . . . in which prostitutes are lodged gregariously, are, generally speaking, under the most complete supervision of the police. Numerous formalities must be gone through before a licence is granted by the *Bureau des Mœurs*, and stringent regulations must be complied with under inexorable penalties. The houses must be confined to the one purpose, excepting in the Banlieue, where, from the impossibility of exercising perfect control, and other considerations, a dispensation is granted to deal, during pleasure, in liquor and tobacco. They may not exist near places of worship, public buildings, schools, furnished hotels, or important factories. They may not be on a common staircase. They are not allowed to be near one another, within the walls, but in the Banlieue their concentration is imposed. They must be distinguished from other houses by the size of the figures of their number, which must be two feet in length. . . .

Among the regulations applicable to the *maîtresses*, or *dames de maison*, are the following:

They must lodge no more inmates than they have distinct rooms;

They may keep no child above four years old upon the premises;

They must report, within twenty-four hours, every application made to them for lodgings, and every change of lodgers, and also keep accurate registers for the inspection of the police. Their windows must be kept constantly closed, and be either of ground glass or provided with blinds and curtains;

They may place no person at their door as a sign of their business, before seven or after eleven, P.M.;

They must enforce upon the women under their authority the observance of the provisions of the *carte*;

They may not receive minors, or students in uniform; and

They must report immediately all cases of disease, and generally keep record of all that passes in their houses, or transpires with regard to their inmates.

Those of the Banlieue must conduct their lodgers once in every week to the central sanitary office for examination; must demand the permits of the military at night, and make return of all cases of excessive expenditure on their premises, or residence by strangers for more than twenty-four hours.

They may not send abroad more than one woman each at one time, the effect of which provision is that there being (for the sake of example) 204 houses and 1,504 *femmes numérotées* on the register, the streets may be said to be permanently secured against the presence of 1,298 individuals of the class.

The *dames de maison* are of course a vicious and, as a general rule, ferocious mercenary band, tyrannizing over the unfortunate helots who form their stock-in-trade, and abjectly crouching before the inspector, the surgeon, and the *mouchard*.* The possession of a house of this kind is the highest aspiration of the prostitute. Such a woman sometimes succeeds in attaining to this pernicious eminence, but it is more frequently in the hands of families in whom houses and goodwill descend as heritable property. The recent editors of Parent's work instance that as much as £2,400 has been given for such an establishment, and £8 has been offered as fine to avoid suspension for three days of one of the lowest. Large as these sums may seem, especially when reduced into francs, they will by no means surprise persons cognizant of the property amassed by those who minister, for ready money only, to the lower gratifications of even our more thrifty countrymen.

The gains of the mistresses of these houses in the better part of Paris are enormous. A medical friend told me that he once, while attending a woman of this class, said he supposed she gained a great deal? – 'Yes, my income is considerable,' she replied, 'more than the pay of a French *maréchal!*'

I have above alluded to the external signs by which these houses may be recognized; they are not unfrequently pointed out to the stranger by the *Laquais de place*, who think that all foreigners are anxious to see them. And certainly the visitor discovers on entering them scenes of sensual extravagance, to which his eyes are unaccustomed in England. Here vice finds a retreat of voluptuous splendour, to which in soberer climes she is a stranger. The visitor is received by the mistress of the house, and ushered into a sumptuous ante-room; on a curtain being drawn aside, a door is revealed to him, containing a circular piece of glass about the size of a crown piece, through which he can reconnoitre at his ease a small, but well-lighted and elegantly-furnished, drawing-room, occupied by the women of the establishment. They are usually to be seen seated on sofa chairs, elegantly attired in different-coloured silks, with low bodies, and having their hair dressed in the extreme of fashion; the whole group being arranged artistically, as in a *tableau vivant*, and the individuals who comprise it representing the poses of different celebrated statues, selected apparently with the object of showing off to the best advantage the peculiar attractions of the different women. From the

* [*mouchard*, detective. See p. 107 below.]

room of observation the visitor can, if he pleases, select his victim, in the same way as the traveller in Galway, on his arrival at a certain hotel, can choose from a number of fish swimming about in the tank the particular salmon on which he would prefer to dine. If this somewhat cold-blooded process of selection is distasteful to him, and he desires to become acquainted with the women in a less summary manner – or if the object of his visit is merely amusement, or the satisfaction of curiosity, without any ulterior aim – he can enter the room, and enjoy the society of its occupants, and will find that the terms of the invitation addressed by the old women at the street door to passers-by are strictly carried out – 'Si vous montez voir les jolies filles cela vous engage à rien',* all that is expected from him being to stand a reasonable amount of champagne, or other refreshment, and make himself generally agreeable. It is almost unnecessary to add that to indulge such curiosity is an act of extreme rashness, for in such places all that is possible is done to rob vice of its hideousness, and the visitor is surrounded by an atmosphere of luxury, and by all accessories calculated to captivate the senses and arouse desire. In some of these houses scenes may be witnessed which can only be enacted by women utterly dead to every sense of shame, in whom every vestige of decency has been trampled out, leaving them merely animated machines, for stimulating and gratifying the basest passions.

The life of these women must be monotonous enough. They rise about ten, breakfast at eleven (*à la fourchette* [a knife-and-fork meal]), dine at half-past five, and sup about two; they seldom go out walking, and when they do it is in the company of the mistress or sub-mistress. They pay great and minute attention to their persons, taking baths very frequently, and spending the greater part of the day between breakfast and dinner in preparing their toilette, gossiping together, and smoking cigarettes; some few can play the piano (an instrument usually to be found in these houses), but, as a rule, they are, as might be expected, totally devoid of accomplishments. They have no rooms to themselves, but live *en pension*, taking their meals together; the mistress of the house, or her husband, or lover, as the case may be, presides, and the women take precedence at table among themselves, according to the time that they have been

* ['You can go up and look at the pretty girls without any obligation.']

in the establishment. After dinner, commences the operation of dressing, and otherwise preparing themselves for the public, who chiefly frequent these houses in the evening, and after midnight. By half-past seven or eight o'clock they are ready to make their appearance immediately on the bell being rung.

They are generally dressed in accordance with the latest fashion in vogue at balls and *soirées*, and leave untried no device of art for improving or supplementing nature, spending large sums of money on cosmetics and perfumery, often dyeing their hair and darkening their eyebrows and eyelashes, and in some cases having sores painted over to conceal them from their medical attendant.

These women are undoubtedly, as a rule, well-fed and well-dressed. There is usually a debtor and creditor account between them and the mistress of the house, with whom it is always an object to keep her lodgers in her debt, this being the only hold she can have upon them. They are supposed, by a pleasing fiction, to pay nothing for their lodging, firing, and light, and there is certainly no actual charge made on this account; but, as a makeweight, one-half of what they earn is considered to be the mistress's portion, while the other half is paid over to these avaricious duennas, and goes towards defraying the boarding and other expenses. Such a bargain can only be struck by utterly improvident and reckless persons, and goes far towards proving them incapable of regulating their expenses for themselves; it is believed in France that, if they were not cared for by their mistresses, they would sink at once into the extreme of poverty, and this affords, to my mind, one of the few excuses that can be made for the toleration of such houses. I have read in a French work upon prostitution some horrid paragraphs that I do not care to extract, showing the fearful depth of infamy to which these miserable women are sunk, it being even hinted that their mistresses compel them to practise unnatural crimes by threats of expulsion, to which also they are encouraged by extra *douceurs* [presents] from the debauched *habitués*. So long as a woman is much sought after, the mistress proves obsequious and kind, taking her occasionally to the theatre, and permitting her other indulgences; but so soon as the public desert the waning prostitute, a cause of quarrel is found, and she is brutally turned out of doors, often with no better covering than an old petticoat or worn-out dress. Thus is it that the public prostitutes step at once from luxurious *salons* to dirty hovels. A man-servant is rarely met with in these houses, the domestics being generally prostitutes.

Parent-Duchâtelet, in speaking of the inmates of these houses, says these unfortunates

> are obliged to abandon themselves to the first comer who calls for them, even if he is covered with the most disgusting sores; there is no drawing back, if they would avoid blows and the very worst treatment. Their mistresses give them no rest; for, to make use of a comparison that has often been employed by the inspectors, the most brutal carter takes greater care of the horses in his charge than these women do of the girls they make a fortune out of.*

The downward course of a prostitute is thus described by Alphonse Esquiros:

> The young, pretty, and pleasant-looking girl starts her career in the better class of houses; but each year, each month makes her less attractive. In a very short time the thermometer goes right down to ugliness. The girl too goes down, from house to house, from indignity to indignity, from district to district. To those who have been unable to shelter themselves from the reverses of their calling, either by putting aside a little money or by providing themselves with a home, the autumn of life brings dreadful suffering. The girl must leave the private room to walk the streets in the rain and cold, half-clothed, looking for that universal and lost husband who elbows her aside. She must submit to the insults and taunts of her younger companions, who are foolish enough to jeer at her decrepitude. Many of these old women are not yet thirty-two. . . . Let a girl once enter these houses, she must necessarily bid farewell to heaven, liberty, honour, and the world. I would write over the door of such a house those celebrated words of the Italian poet: 'All hope abandon, ye who enter here.'†

The houses appropriated in Paris to the temporary accommodation of prostitutes and their frequenters, termed *maisons de passe*, have been always considered more dangerous to public morality than the mere lodging-houses. They have been consequently the

---

* [Parent-Duchâtelet, *De la prostitution dans la ville de Paris*, 3rd edition (1857), I. 681–2. Acton's translation has been slightly amended.]

† [Esquiros, *Les Vierges folles*, 3rd edition (1842), 117–18, 80. Acton's translation has been amended.]

objects of much anxious vigilance by the authorities, who, nevertheless, proceeding on the principle that anything is preferable to uncontrolled clandestine prostitution, have taken them under their supervision so far as possible. Their numbers are, however, unknown. The only record given by Parent, and we may therefore safely assume the only one to be got, is, that in 1825 there were 150 of them recognized. To facilitate the operation of the police, every such establishment is compelled to bear on its books two registered women, and is therefore to all intents and purposes subject to the general dispositions with regard to the *maisons publiques*. The proprietors are subject to heavy penalties for receiving, *en passe*, girls under fifteen years of age, public women not known to them, or verified as such by production of the *carte*, or students of the public schools.

The *fille en carte* of Paris obtains, of course, what she can for her services, but the usual fee is from two to five francs. In the tolerated houses, the sum charged by the establishment varies from five to twenty, in addition to which the generosity of the visitor usually dictates a trifling present to the victim, *pour ses gants* [glove-money], as it is called. At the Barriers, artisans pay by custom one franc, soldiers fifty centimes, or a fivepenny silver piece. Excited to drink (for, as I have mentioned, the sale of liquor at the lowest class of houses is winked at by the police) by their visitors and the *dames de maison*, each from different motives, these *filles numérotées* of the Banlieue are from habitual intoxication so incapable of sanitary precautions or observance of decorum, that in their case, at least, the regulations of the *Bureau des Mœurs* may be esteemed rather a blessing than a curse.

Similar systems, more or less improved upon the Parisian type, prevail at Toulon, Lyons, Strasburg, Brest, and other large French garrison towns. . . .

This sketch of French prostitution would be incomplete if I did not compare the condition of the streets of Paris with that of our own. The prostitutes in Paris are not spread over all the streets, as in London; they are only to be found in certain localities prescribed by the police. The *fille de maison* may be met gaudily dressed, quickly walking backwards and forwards, in certain back streets; but even there she is not allowed to actually solicit, though, as may be supposed, she does not fail to attract the attention of passers-by.

The *fille à carte* is the prostitute whom the stranger is most likely to meet with, and she is generally less gaudily dressed than the *fille de maison*, and is allowed by the police to walk up and down in certain less frequented streets, but not to go beyond them. She likewise is not allowed to solicit.

The clandestine prostitute, notwithstanding all the precautions of the police to register every woman gaining her livelihood by prostitution, is frequently to be met with in the streets of Paris. Work girls, servants, and girls serving in shops, who wish to increase their small earnings, and yet are not registered by the police, come under the head of clandestine prostitutes. These last of course are not more subject to control than ordinary persons, but the police in Paris strictly supervise all women known by them to be prostitutes, and render the streets passable at all hours of the evening or night to respectable females, and solicitation is strictly forbidden. Moreover, Frenchmen do not, as a rule, go into the streets of Paris after dinner to meet with adventures; they rather frequent the casinos or houses of accommodation. And even if some women are to be seen in certain streets in Paris in the early part of the evening, after half-past eleven the streets are quite deserted, as the police oblige every woman to retire to her room at that hour. How different is the condition of the streets of London; and we might well follow in this respect the example of the French. In London a man has prostitution thrust upon him; in Paris he has to go out of his way to look for it; so that external decency, so outraged in England, is there maintained.

*   *   *

There are, I believe, thirty detectives employed in Paris to watch and trace clandestine prostitutes. If they see a suspicious-looking woman in the streets or at the public balls, they follow and arrest her, and unless she can give a satisfactory account of herself, she is examined, and if found diseased, sent to the St Lazare Hospital, three francs being the premium paid for her discovery. These *mouchards*, as they are called, become as well known to the women as a hawk is to small birds. I was present on one occasion when some captured women arrived at the hospital. They were brought like prisoners in an omnibus, which was driven into the courtyard. I was given to understand they were fair representatives of their class; if so, they are very plain. The women whom I saw on this occasion were short and thickset, but not altogether unprepossessing; although generally stout, they did not look as if they drank freely, nor were they sensuous-looking, but all the police authorities agree that they would rather gain their subsistence by prostitution than work. Idleness is their besetting sin. On the occasion I refer to, they appeared to consider their calling like any other occupation, and to regard one another with an *esprit de corps*, as if they were so many postmen or policemen – prudery and impudence were equally absent. They seemed only anxious to escape from captivity, which they could not do without the signature of the medical man, certifying that they were sound. They appeared to treat the contagious diseases with which they were infected as so many evils incidental to their business. Every profession has its drawbacks! I was told that it is mostly the young girls who are diseased; the older prostitutes avoid contagion by examining every man who desires to have relations with them, previously to permitting intercourse; but these even are not exempt from uterine affections, and suffer seriously from the complaints peculiar to their sex, quite independently of venereal disease.

The object of the wary, old prostitute is to exercise her calling with the least expenditure of self, and to gain as much money as possible. In reply to my question, why do so many old, deformed, and worn-out women carry on the *métier* [profession] and not retire, I was told that to live required food, and to gain the wherewithal to appease their appetites for luxuries entailed labour – now these women prefer prostituting their persons to gaining a livelihood by honest labour, and seem to think that they are not humiliated thereby, but regard themselves as a class useful to the State and recognized by the police. And notwithstanding what the public may think, they do not despise themselves till they are worn out, when they gradually pass into some other calling. Those whom I saw did not look vicious, but seemed well to do in the world, and so far as I could judge, were not much troubled with aught else than how to live from hand to mouth. In only one instance at this examination at which I assisted was any feeling of modesty evinced, one woman objecting to the presence of anyone but the regular medical attendant; however, when told that I was a foreign doctor, she seemed quite satisfied. All the others entered, and were examined as if it formed part of the day's duty.

★ ★ ★

The women whom I saw [at the Lourcine Hospital] were very cleanly, and although at the examination at which I assisted there were at least fifty of them brought promiscuously from different parts of Paris, it was not found necessary to send one to the hospital. Few of these women were good-looking, and most of them appeared to be middle-aged, and one who, I should think, was sixty years of age, was, to my surprise, still on the register. I had some suspicion as to the cause of her appearance in such company, as she could hardly have been carrying on the trade on her own account; she was probably an agent in the pay of one of the houses – half spy, half procuress. I asked one crooked-eyed woman who came from the suburbs of Paris, how many men she was accustomed to receive per day; she replied, ten or twelve. The fee paid her by soldiers was usually half a franc, other men paying a franc. On being further questioned, this woman admitted that she sometimes received as many as forty men in twenty-four hours. Notwithstanding such excesses as these, the generative organs presented no unusual appearances. I, however, pass by the other questions I put to these women, to describe a circumstance unprecedented in the whole of my previous or subsequent inquiries on this painful subject. A girl about seventeen, possessing a good figure, and very intelligent, was introduced, looking frightened and abashed. 'Doctor,' said she, 'I am truly in distress; I have nothing to eat; see the rags which cover me. I have received a fair education, but have been turned out of house and home. I have, I acknowledge, an inherited impetuous temper, and poverty compels me to come here. I am about to enter on a life of infamy, but no other course is open to me. I hope you will find me sound. I know I am not diseased, for I have never known man. Wicked as I am, I have done all in my power to be again received at home, and I desire to enter Madame ——'s house.' The police, before inscribing such a girl on the public register, and introducing her to prostitution, would write to her parents. She underwent the examination, was declared sound, and existence, at least, was thus assured to her for a time.

I am not aware that any system in any civilized country exists which could prevent such a girl taking such a course. She passed from my sight, but has left on my mind an indelible impression, and I insert the sad story here, believing that its recital may bring home to the reader, in the most forcible manner possible, the full horrors of prostitution.

Do many prostitutes, we may well ask, enter upon their career in this way? Is their name legion? Who shall say?

★   ★   ★

FRENCH MILITARY AND NAVAL EXPERIENCE

It would appear . . . that [in 1865] the effective force of the French Army consisted of 348,968 men. During that year, 31,918 soldiers suffered from venereal diseases; hence it follows that 92 per 1,000 men only are affected, instead of 325, the average number among English troops. . . . We must admit that venereal diseases are nearly four times more common among our troops than they are among the French. Dr Jeannel says the treatment of venereal patients in the French forces, both by land and sea, costs annually £60,000; the treatment of venereal patients costs the civil hospitals of Paris alone more than £24,000. This sum must be quadrupled if we wish to appreciate the expense required by the treatment of civil venereal patients in the whole of France.

It may then be affirmed that in France venereal diseases cause hospital annual expenses to amount to £156,000 at the least.

If, as seen in previous pages, the authorities in France have found it desirable to legislate for the prostitute, the army has not been forgotten, and precautions have been taken to protect the French soldier from the consequences of prostitution, and the regulations are very strictly carried out in France.

Every French soldier or sailor attacked with syphilis is bound to report himself to the surgeon-major of the service to which he belongs, and should he do so spontaneously, receives no punishment. If he should not do so, he is . . . punished with a month *de consigne* [confined to barracks] on his leaving hospital. He is called upon to point out the woman that has infected him; but this regulation is hard to enforce, as, rather than inform, the men take punishment. In many cases it would be an impossibility, as they frequent a plurality of women, and are occasionally too far gone in liquor at the time of the act to establish an identity.

Every soldier, sailor, or workman in the arsenals is, moreover, subjected, on his arrival at his station, to a special examination; and if any traces of syphilis, however slight, are detected, he is immediately sent to hospital. The more trifling venereal affections are, however, treated at the barracks, a circumstance deserving, I think, the attention of the home authorities in England, who send every case, however slight, to hospital. The penalties which formerly were in vogue when a man was found diseased, are now never inflicted, unless the culprit has attempted to evade the ordinary examination. No one is granted leave of absence without previously undergoing an examination, whereby his freedom from contagious disease may be ascertained.

★ ★ ★

From the discoveries made with regard to clandestine prostitution in France and other Continental countries, we learn the evils to which the prostitutes in this country must, of necessity, be exposed, and which they must as surely entail on the community. They are in a few words at once the victims and the vehicles of loathsome disease, and are exposed to the most cruel and abject misery. The public prostitutes on the Continent are, as we have seen, free to a great extent from the disease, and present it when existing in a mitigated form. The advocates of public prostitution are not necessarily seeking to introduce the terrible *maisons de filles*. We see from the example of Berlin that brothels are not necessary adjuncts to the public system. To create and maintain a class of harlots for the benefit of the public health is, doubtless, repugnant to English feelings, and to preserve public decency by licensing vice, seems to us an intolerable outrage on religion. Such a system appears better suited to heathen times, and to grate harshly on Christian civilization; it has, however, at least, the merit of being logical, and is, apart from its cruelty, in accordance with common sense. It sees an evil, and, therefore, seeks a remedy – a dire disease, and, therefore, withstands its progress and limits its sphere of action – a vice incurable, irrepressible, and, therefore, seeks to regulate it; unfortunately the method adopted has, at least, the appearance of sanctioning vice, and undoubtedly tends to harden the heart and to blunt the conscience. While remembering the injury it inflicts on individuals, we cannot but admire the benefits that it bestows on the public, and from a material point of view, even on its victims.

Nor must we shut our eyes to the plentiful provision that French charity, with which its cruelty is so strangely discordant, makes for the relief of the suffering. We are wont to be proud of the exuberance of English bounty; in this instance, at all events, our neighbours put us to the blush. The French system, though fairly obnoxious to the charge of sacrificing the individual to the public, is careful, so far as it can, to provide relief for the sufferings that it creates or finds, and with all its inherent mischief may compare favourably with the dull stupidity that shuts its eyes to well-known evils, and by refusing to recognize accomplished facts and actual circumstances, endows them with a tenfold power of mischief, and which, while it justifies its inertness by religious theories, forgets the first practical duty of the Christian, which is, to 'love his neighbour as himself', or, in other words, never to be made aware of the miseries of others without attempting, if he has the power, to provide a remedy. And thus starting from false premises, though with the best intention, Christian England persistently neglects to heal the sick, to raise the fallen, or to elevate the morals of the people, and not only provides a plentiful supply of evil for the present, but lays up for the future still more abundant mischief. We may be assured that all the evils found on the Continent to be inseparably linked with clandestine prostitution, are present with ourselves in at least an equal degree. Would we know what is English prostitution, we may find it if we will not search at home reflected accurately in clandestine prostitution abroad. From what has been done in foreign lands, we may learn what might be done at home, and the evils into which others have fallen – in the honest effort from which we shrink at home to provide a remedy for the worst form of human misery – should be regarded not so much as rocks on which we must inevitably strike and sink, as beacons to warn us of the dangers into which others have fallen, and to enable us to avoid them.

6

CAUSES OF PROSTITUTION

I HAVE to the best of my ability called attention to prostitution as existing among us in the present day, by laying before the reader such facts as I have been able to gather concerning it both in this and other countries. We may now, informed as to the nature of the evil with which we have to deal, and guided by the experience gained in foreign lands, consider what measures we can best adopt for alleviating the evils incident to it, and for checking, so far as possible, the system itself.

It seems not inconvenient at the outset of such a discussion to consider the causes that produce, or tend to perpetuate, the evil state of things with which we have in the previous chapters become acquainted. Such an inquiry may at first appear superfluous, for unhappily these causes are neither few nor far to seek, and only too apparent to the most careless observer. It will, however, become evident on reflection, that a mere indistinct appreciation of them is not sufficient for our purpose, which requires a distinct and methodical statement, setting the different causes under their appropriate heads, and thus enabling us to separate those inherent to human life, and ineradicable, from those dependent on accident and circumstance, and capable of diminution, if not of removal. Practical legislation on a difficult and intricate subject, which requires careful and delicate handling, is the object before us – the more plain, simple, and unambitious the legislation, the greater chance will there be of its proving successful. Sentimental and utopian schemes must be avoided; the line between the possible and the impossible clearly drawn; existing facts and the conclusions fairly deducible from them, however painful, must be recognized, to enable us to do this and to produce a plain, straightforward, and practical remedy for the very serious evils depicted in my earlier chapters. We must clearly appreciate not only the effect, but the cause.

I may first of all broadly state the somewhat self-evident

proposition that prostitution exists, and flourishes, because there is a demand for the article supplied by its agency.

Supply, as we all know, is regulated by demand, and demand is the practical expression of an ascertained want. Want and demand may be either natural or artificial. Articles necessary for the support, or protection of life, such as meat, and drink, fire, clothes, and lodging, are the objects of natural demand. In these the extent of the demand is measured entirely by the want, and this latter will neither be increased by an abundance of supply, nor diminished by a scarcity. Articles of luxury are the objects of artificial demand, which depends not merely on the want, but is actually increased by the supply; that is to say, the desire for these articles grows with the possession and enjoyment of them. This feature is peculiarly noticeable in prostitution, though in strictness, perhaps, it cannot be placed in the category of artificial wants. The want of prostitutes grows with the use of them. We may also observe that in other cases the demand is active, and the supply passive, in this the supply is active, so that we may almost say the supply rather than the want creates the demand.

We must not here lose sight of the fact that the desire for sexual intercourse is strongly felt by the male on attaining puberty, and continues through his life an ever-present, sensible want; it is most necessary to keep this in view, for, true though it be, it is constantly lost sight of, and erroneous theories, producing on the one hand coercive legislation, on the other neglect of obvious evils, are the result. This desire of the male is the want that produces the demand, of which prostitution is a result, and which is, in fact, the artificial supply of a natural demand, taking the place of the natural supply through the failure of the latter, or the vitiated character of the demand. It is impossible to exaggerate the force of sexual desire. We must, however, bear in mind that man is not a mere material existence; his nature includes also mind and spirit, and he is endowed with conscience to admonish, reason to regulate, and will to control his desires and actions. Woman was created to be the companion of man, and her nature presents the exact counterpart of his. It is evident, that if so composite a being permits any of the different constituent parts of his nature to attain to undue proportions, he thereby impoverishes and weakens the others, and in proportion as he does this, and accords indulgence to one set of qualities and inclinations at the expense of the rest, he deteriorates from his real nature. He is, in truth, an unmanly man, who devotes all his time and care to athletic and physical pursuits and enjoyments. So is the man who forgets or despises his body, and gives all his care to the mind and intellect. And so also is the man who withdraws from life its enjoyments and duties, and devotes himself exclusively to meditation and spiritual exercise. Men, in proportion as the different elements in their being receive fair play and produce their desires, may be considered to approach more or less nearly the standard of human perfection.

The intercourse, therefore, of man or woman ought to appeal to their threefold organization of body, mind, and spirit. If the first predominates over and excludes the others, sexual desire degenerates into lust; when all are present, it is elevated into love, which appeals to each of the component parts of man's nature. The men who seek gratification for, and the women who bestow it on, one part of their being only are in an unnatural state. And here we may distinguish the indulgence of unlawful love from commerce with prostitutes, the one is the ill-regulated but complete gratification of the entire human being, the other affords gratification to one part only of his nature.

One other distinction also we must carefully notice, and that is that in the one case the enjoyment is mutual, and that in the other the enjoyment is one-sided, and granted not as the expression and reward of love, but as a matter of commerce. But if it be derogatory to their being, and unnatural to bestow gratification on one part of their nature only, what shall we say of the condition of those unfortunate women to whom sexual indulgence affords no pleasure, and who pass their lives in, and gain their living by, affording enjoyments which they do not share, and feigning a passion which has ceased to move them? The woman who abandons herself for gain, instead of in obedience to the promptings of desire – who,

> while her Lover pants upon her breast,
> Can mark the figures on an Indian chest; * –

is in an unnatural state, and so is the man who uses her, and obtains for a mere money consideration that enjoyment of the person which

* [Pope, *Epistles to Several Persons* (*Moral Essays*), ii. 167–9. Acton misquotes, substituting 'count' for Pope's 'mark'.]

should be yielded only as the result and crowning expression of mutual passion. We may further observe that commerce with a prostitute is an ephemeral transaction, which (though it may be followed by serious consequences) yet entails no obligations. Illicit attachments are more lasting, though usually transitory, and entail limited obligations. Both conditions are substitutes for, or imitations of the relationship resulting from love, and known as the married state, which, arising from mutual desire, and granting the highest privileges, imposes corresponding obligations, and is usually as lasting as life itself, and proves at once the mainspring and chief safeguard of society.

We may now consider a little more in detail the want, the demand, and the supply. The want is, in its inception, a natural want, and is simply the perversion of the natural desire of every male for female companionship; it is asserted by some writers that indulgence in sexual intercourse is necessary for the male as soon as he has attained puberty, and they present us with pitiable pictures of the unhappy condition to which many are reduced, who from timidity or religious or moral influences refrain from giving free scope to their desires, and who deduce from this the somewhat startling proposition that freer sexual intercourse than is at present countenanced by the conscience and practice of society, should be accorded. No doubt the cases cited by the supporters of this theory are very pitiable; they will, however, scarcely have the hardihood to assert that marriage immediately on attaining puberty would tend to the proper development of the man, or be otherwise than injurious. Rather than marriage or sexual gratification, we would suggest, as the true remedy, that morbid excitement should be corrected by healthy bodily exercise and mental application. If the young permit themselves to dwell unduly on sexual ideas a demoralized condition of mind and body must result. For helpless sufferers, if such there are, and their existence be not simply due to the imagination of prejudiced advocates of immorality and wickedness, the cure is to be found in the cricket-field, the river, or the racquet-court, and the different athletic sports and intellectual studies suitable to their age. I confidently assert that marriage or sexual indulgence, before maturity is attained, is most prejudicial.

To show that abstinence is not in itself injurious, the case of the ancient Germans may be cited, to whom the company of the other sex was strictly prohibited until their age had exceeded twenty years. Their stalwart frames and reckless valour were the admiration and terror of the more dissolute Romans, to whose well-armed and disciplined legions their naked prowess opposed a long, doubtful conflict; their vigorous bodies, martial countenances, and intrepid conduct, proved that abstinence from sexual indulgence had neither tamed their spirit nor weakened their physique. It may be objected that the times with which we have to do are more artificial, and that it is impossible for the boy to emerge into youth and manhood without having sexual ideas presented to his mind. The difference is one only of degree. Let him eschew sexual thoughts and obscene conversation, and give himself to healthy exercise and vigorous study, and sexual abstinence, far from proving injurious, will scarcely seem a hardship.

This position is further strengthened by the analogy of the lower creation. Stallions are not put too early to the stud. The rams reserved till two years old produce a better progeny than those employed for this purpose at one year old. Bulls may be used at nine months, but those destined to perpetuate the short-horn and other valuable breeds are permitted first to attain the age of two years. So much for the natural want. The want that finds relief in prostitutes, is the unbridled desire of precocious youths and vicious men. In like manner, the demand is occasioned by the indulgence of the vicious, and therefore unnatural, want. It arises from men forgetting that they are not placed in this world merely to gratify their appetites. Life has its lawful pleasures; it has also its duties and obligations. Idleness is easier than industry, but the rewards of life are given to the diligent. . . . To steal is easier than to work, self-indulgence than self-restraint. . . . Man's plain duty is to seek in honourable love the gratification of manly desire, and to wait for enjoyment till he has earned the right to it. 'Be fruitful and multiply, and replenish the earth,' is the Divine reason for the presence of the sexual instinct. 'Flee youthful lusts,' the Divine rule of life. There is a right and wrong way of gratifying natural desires: it is, as we have seen, not only possible to choose the right, but more beneficial both to mind and body. . . .

The demand for prostitution arises, then, from ill-regulated and uncontrolled desire, and may be referred to the following heads:

The natural instinct of man.

His sinful nature.

The artificial state of society rendering early marriages difficult if not impossible.

The unwillingness of many, who can afford marriage, to submit to its restraint, and incur its obligations.

To a man's calling preventing him from marrying, or debarring him when married from conjugal intercourse.

The unrestrained want and lawless demand, call for the infamous supply; but want and demand are insufficient of themselves to create supply; there are strong provoking causes, but not creative. We must go a step further to discover the sources of supply. It is derived from the vice of women, which is occasioned by:

Natural desire.

Natural sinfulness.

The preferment of indolent ease to labour.

Vicious inclinations strengthened and ingrained by early neglect, or evil training, bad associates, and an indecent mode of life.

Necessity, imbued by

The inability to obtain a living by honest means consequent on a fall from virtue.

Extreme poverty.

To this black list may be added love of drink, love of dress, love of amusement, while the fall from virtue may result either from a woman's love being bestowed on an unworthy object, who fulfils his professions of attachment by deliberately accomplishing her ruin, or from the woman's calling peculiarly exposing her to temptation. . . .

Prostitution is at once a result produced by and a cause producing immorality. Every unchaste woman is not a prostitute. By unchastity a woman becomes liable to lose character, position, and the means of living; and when these are lost is too often reduced to prostitution for support, which, therefore, may be described as the trade adopted by all women who have abandoned or are precluded from an honest course of life, or who lack the power or the inclination to obtain a livelihood from other sources. What is a prostitute? She is a woman who gives for money that which she ought to give only for love; who ministers to passion and lust alone, to the exclusion and extinction of all the higher qualities, and nobler sources of enjoyment which combine with desire, to produce the happiness derived from the

CAUSES OF PROSTITUTION

intercourse of the sexes. She is a woman with half the woman gone,
and that half containing all that elevates her nature, leaving her a
mere instrument of impurity; degraded and fallen she extracts from
the sin of others the means of living, corrupt and dependent on
corruption, and therefore interested directly in the increase of immorality – a social pest, carrying contamination and foulness to every
quarter to which she has access, who,

> like a ... disease, ...
> Creeps, no precaution used, among the crowd,
> Makes wicked lightnings of her eyes, ...
> ... and stirs the pulse,
> With devil's leaps, and poisons half the young.*

Such women, ministers of evil passions, not only gratify desire, but
also arouse it. Compelled by necessity to seek for customers, they
throng out streets and public places, and suggest evil thoughts and
desires which might otherwise remain undeveloped. Confirmed
profligates will seek out the means of gratifying their desires; the
young from a craving to discover unknown mysteries may approach
the haunts of sin, but thousands would remain uncontaminated if
temptation did not seek them out. Prostitutes have the power of
soliciting and tempting. Gunpowder remains harmless till the spark
falls upon it; the match, until struck, retains the hidden fire, so lust
remains dormant till called into being by an exciting cause.

The sexual passion is strong in every man, but it is strong in proportion as it is encouraged or restrained; and every act of indulgence
only makes future abstinence more hard, and in time almost impossible. Some consider that prostitution is the safety valve of society,
and that any serious diminution of the number of prostitutes would
be attended with an increase of clandestine immodesty. Such a consequence is not one that I think need be apprehended; the insinua-
tion that virtuous women, to be made to yield, require only to be
assaulted, is a base and unworthy calumny; nor is it to be supposed
that the man who will use a harlot is prepared to insult or injure a
modest woman. But intercourse with depraved women debases the
mind, and gradually hardens the heart, and each act of gratification
stimulates desire and necessitates fresh indulgence; and when

* [Tennyson, *Idylls of the King* (1859), 'Guinevere', ll. 514–18.]

grown into a habit, not only breeds distaste for virtuous society, but causes the mind to form a degraded estimate of the sex, until all women seem mere objects of desire and vehicles of indulgence. The prostitute is a sad burlesque of woman, presenting herself as an object of lust instead of an object of honourable love – a source of base gratification, instead of a reason for self-restraint; familiarizing man with this aspect of women till he can see no other, and his indulged body and debased mind lead him to seek in them only sensual gratification, and to make, if possible, of every woman the thing that he desires – a toy, a plaything, an animated doll; a thing to wear like a glove, and fling away; to use like a horse, and send to the knackers when worn out; the mere object of his fancy and servant of his appetite, instead of an immortal being, composed, like himself, of body, soul and spirit – his associate and consort, endowed with memory and hope and strong affections, with a heart to love, to feel, to suffer; man's highest prize and surest safeguard; the inspirer of honest love and manly exertion, powerful

> Not only to keep down the base in man,
> But teach high thought, and amiable words
> And courtliness, and the desire of fame,
> And love of truth, and all that makes a man.*

It thus appears that prostitution depends not only on demand and supply, and external causes, but is itself a cause of its own existence, because the possibility of indulgence weakens the force of self-restraint, by creating the idea in the mind of unlawfully and basely gratifying the natural instinct, to which indulgence adds force and intensity, and thus in a measure creates the want, producing from a desire capable of restraint a habit impossible to shake off. While the supply being active, and itself desiring exercise, does not wait for the demand, but goes about to seek it, suggesting, arousing, stimulating evil thoughts and unhallowed passions. . . .

The divine command, 'Be fruitful, and multiply and replenish the earth' . . . is the law of our being, and our instincts accord with the law. It is impossible, therefore, that the sexual passion can ever die out, nor is it to be desired that it should; so long as it continues, however, prostitution is at least possible.

* [*Ibid.* ll. 476–9.]

The children of Adam not only possess this instinct – they have also a sinful nature, which is as much a part of their being as the natural instinct: the one is as ineradicable as the other, and so long as this natural instinct remains allied with a sinful nature, human beings will be liable to be dragged into impurity and unlawful indulgence, and so long as they remain in this condition prostitution is inevitable. . . .

I consider it would be alike ungenerous to attempt to paraphrase, and impossible to express better than himself, the ideas of 'Theophrastus', upon the anti-matrimonial tendencies of modern middle-class society, in his communication entitled, 'The Other Side of the Picture', to the editor of *The Times*, May 7, 1857:

The laws which society imposes in the present day in respect of marriage upon young men belonging to the middle class are, in the highest degree, unnatural, and are the real cause of most of our social corruptions. The father of a family has, in many instances, risen from a comparatively humble origin to a position of easy competence. His wife has her carriage; he associates with men of wealth greater than his own. His sons reach the age when, in the natural course of things, they ought to marry and establish a home for themselves. It would seem no great hardship that a young couple should begin on the same level as their parents began, and be content for the first few years with the mere necessaries of life; and there are thousands who, were it not for society, would gladly marry on such terms. But here the tyrant world interposes; the son must not marry until he can maintain an establishment on much the same footing as his father's. If he dare to set the law at defiance, his family lose caste, and he and his wife are quietly dropt out of the circle in which they have hitherto moved. All that society will allow is an engagement, and then we have the sad but familiar sight of two young lovers wearing out their best years with hearts sickened with hope long deferred; often, after all, ending in disappointment, or in the shattered health of the poor girl, unable to bear up against the harassing anxiety. Or even when a long engagement does finally end in marriage, how diminished are the chances of happiness. The union, which, if allowed at first, would have proved happy under worldly difficulty, has lost its brightness when postponed until middle life, even with competence and a carriage. Perhaps the early struggles would have only strengthened the bonds of affection; but here I feel that I am on dangerous ground. Already I hear society loudly exclaiming that I am advocating improvident marriages, that I would flood the country with genteel paupers, that I am advising what is contrary to the best interests of society

But stay awhile, society. Your picture of marriages at thirty-five, with a Belgravian house for the happy couple, a footman in splendid uniform, and at least a brougham, is very pleasing; but there is a reverse to the canvas, and that a very dark one. How has the bridegroom been living since he attained his manhood? I believe that there are very many young men who are keeping themselves pure amid all the temptations of London life. God's blessing be with them, for they are the salt of our corrupt city. But I know that there are thousands who are living in sin, chiefly in consequence of the impossibility (as the world says) of their marrying. Some go quietly with the stream, and do as others do around them, almost without a thought of the misery they are causing, and the curse they are laying up for themselves. But many, perhaps most of them, are wretched under the convictions of their conscience. Living in the midst of temptation, they have not sufficient principle to resist its fascination, and although they know where God intends that they shall find their safety, yet they dare not offend their family, alienate their friends, and lose their social position by making what the world calls an imprudent marriage. The very feeling which Heaven has given as a chief purifier of man's nature is darkening their conscience and hardening their heart, because the law of society contradicts the law of God. I might touch upon even a more terrible result of the present state of things – medical men and clergymen will understand what I mean – but I dare not, and I have said enough.

I must in sadness confess that in the face of the powerful tyranny of social law in this country, it is difficult to suggest any general remedy for this evil. But the mischief is on the increase with our increasing worship of money, and public attention ought to be appealed to on the subject. If our American eulogist be right in commending 'pluck' as one of our distinctive characteristics, it is not our young men who should lack the quality. If they will shake off the affectations of club life, and claim a position in society for themselves and for their wives, because they are qualified for it by education and character, and not merely because they represent so much money, they will soon force the world to give way, and strike down one of the greatest hindrances to their own happiness, both temporal and eternal. It will not in general be difficult to bring the daughters over to the same opinion. Mothers and sisters are seldom very hard-hearted in such cases, and by united efforts the stern father may be induced to give his blessing, even though the happy couple (ay, happy, let the world sneer as it will) have to begin on little more than the proverbial bread and cheese.

The recognition of this principle would do much to check some of our most deadly social evils. It would make many a girl whom the tyranny of the world now dooms to a joyless celibacy a happy wife and mother. It would raise the tone of character of our young men, bringing out into healthful exercise the home affections, which are now denied them, at the very time of life when their influence is most beneficial. It would drive away all frivolity and effeminacy before the realities of steady work, which early marriage would oblige them to face. It would purify our streets, and check many a bitter pang of conscience, and save many a soul. We are experiencing the bitter fruits of man's law – let us see whether God's law will not work better.

The upper ten thousand too often, I fear, forget that the outside million – among whom, it has been quaintly said, they 'condescend to live' – cannot be relied on to travel for ever in the grooves cut out for them by their betters, and assume that if no overt and organized resistance to the Medo-Persian ukases of society and fashion appears on the surface, those edicts are immutable – that tyranny permanent. But the fact is – and they should be reminded of it – that with regard to some things, and among them marriage, there is a numerous and increasing class, by no means the waifs and strays of the community, who are disposed, not to question or propose any change in the law, but simply to ignore it, and to 'put up', as they say, 'with the consequences'.

The numberless cases of *mésalliance* daily occurring, whereof the majority entail, beside the paltry consequence of 'Coventry', the very serious ones of unfruitfulness and domestic infelicity, seem to me to point the finger of warning to the guardians of our social code. That finger indicates a blot upon the table of the law – cause of a nascent canker, which – not, perhaps, for many a long day, but certainly some day – if left untreated, will corrupt the fabric.

I extract the following passages from the admirable editorial remarks upon the foregoing letter of 'Theophrastus':

Do we not make difficulties for ourselves here, even where nature makes none, and create by our system a huge mass of artificial temptation which need never have existed? . . . A great law of Providence cannot be neglected with impunity, and this undue, artificial, and unnatural postponement of marriage ends in a great blot upon our social system. Vice is the result, and vice creates a class of victims to indulge it. If Providence has ordained that man should not live alone, and if conventional maxims or mere empty fashion and the artificial attractions of society lead to overlooking, or superseding, or tampering with this law, the neglect of a Providential law will surely avenge itself in social disease and corruption in one or other part of the system. It is not, then, because we wish for a moment to encourage improvident marriages, but because we feel convinced that our modern caution here has outstepped all reasonable limits, has become extravagant, has from being a dictate of natural common sense become a mere conventional and artificial rule, the voice of empty fashion, and a gratuitous hindrance to social happiness and the designs of Providence, that we call serious attention to this subject. The fear of poverty has become morbid, and men cry out not only before they are hurt, but before there is any reasonable prospect of it. They must see in married life a perfectly guaranteed and undisturbed vista of the amplest pecuniary resources before they will enter upon it. They forget that married men can *work*, and that marriage is a stimulus to work, and again and again elicits those latent activities of mind which produce not only competency, but affluence.*

But, from present signs, so sadly do I, with 'Theophrastus', despair of any contraction, by the lawgivers of fashion, of the ample line of *chevaux de frise* [wire entanglements] they have skilfully disposed round lawful wedlock; so ferocious, on the contrary, is the struggle for 'position', so terrible an Ægis lurks in the bitter sound of 'genteel beggary', that I am more inclined to look for the sanction by society of self-immolation by superfluous virgins, the revival of convents, or the Malthusian modes of checking population which prevail elsewhere, than for the rich, still less the poor genteel, to permit

* *The Times*, May 9, 1857.

their unfeesimpled or undowered offspring to increase and multiply young, so-called 'paupers', of still less estate, without the fear of mammon's law before their eyes, and in obedience to the will of Him who feeds the young ravens.

The foregoing remarks apply, of course, almost exclusively to the upper sections of society, but hindrances to marriage are not confined to the upper classes. I am, however, only concerned with this fact, that by the unwritten custom of society, persons must not marry unless they be in possession of a certain income. We may be thankful that the ecclesiastical law forbidding the clergy to marry, and thereby letting loose on the community thousands of men in danger and adding to the numbers of the tempters and tempted, is no longer in force in this country; still we have some among us whose calling virtually prohibits them from marrying – I allude, of course, to soldiers.

The married establishment of the non-commissioned officers and rank and file of the regiments and corps serving at home and abroad (India excepted), is not permitted to exceed the following proportions:

Our Regimental Staff Sergeants

3 out of	4 or 5		⎫	
4 „	6 „ 7		⎬ Serjeants of each troop, battery,	
5 „	8 „ 9		⎪ or company.	
6 „	10 „ upwards		⎭	

Seven per cent of trumpeters, drummers, and rank and file calculated upon the establishment.

A soldier must have completed seven years' service, and be in possession of at least one good-conduct badge, in order to be eligible to have his name placed on the roll (of married men). Thus we find that 93 out of every 100 soldiers are of necessity unmarried men, and this brings me naturally to my second subdivision, namely, local causes. Considering that the men subject to the above restrictions are for the most part in the prime of life, in vigorous health, and exposed to circumstances peculiarly calculated to develop animal instincts, we may reasonably expect to find a large demand for prostitutes in all garrison towns, and may feel sure that there is always a supply in proportion to the demand. Our principal seaport towns are, of course, exposed to the same evil, from a similar cause.

But prostitution abounds not only in places where large numbers of unmarried men are collected together, but also where in the course of their daily work the sexes are brought into close and intimate relations. Factory towns, therefore, must be included in the list of places peculiarly liable to the presence of prostitution, though perhaps in this case the prevailing mischief may be more accurately termed general immorality, or depravity, than prostitution proper; the difference, however, is not very great, and, for the purposes of this work, immaterial.

I must not forget to include among local causes the serious mischief incidental to the gang system in various agricultural districts. Public attention has on several recent occasions been prominently called to the evils thus arising, and it is not unreasonable to hope that adequate steps will be taken for improving the moral condition of the agricultural poor. Where women and men, and girls and boys are working together indiscriminately in the fields, with, in many cases, long distances to traverse in going to and returning from the scenes of their labours, it is obvious that opportunity cannot be wanting, and that temptations must not infrequently be yielded to, and that the morals and habits of the people will be of a very low order.

We may, however, expect to find large cities contribute in a greater degree than other places to the manufacture and employment of prostitutes. Here always abound idle and wealthy men, with vicious tastes, which they spare neither pains nor expense to gratify. Here also are the needy, the improvident, and the ill-instructed, from whose ranks the victims of sensuality may be readily recruited. The close proximity of luxury and indigence cannot fail to produce a demoralizing effect upon the latter. Garrison, seaport, and factory towns, and large cities, are all places peculiarly liable to the presence of prostitution, containing, as they do, within themselves in an eminent degree the seeds and causes of vice. Some places, such as London, combine within themselves all these qualities, and are therefore notably and exceptionally exposed to this evil. It is impossible to suppose that in such localities prostitution can ever become extinct. Wherever men are peculiarly exposed to temptation by the State, it seems only just that the State should take care that the evil condition that it imposes should be rendered as little injurious as possible. This position has of late years, as we have seen, received a tardy recognition; it is reasonable, I think, to extend this principle a little further, and to adopt a similar course in all cases where we know that the existence of vice is inevitable; it is useless to shut our eyes to a fact; it is better to recognize it – to regulate the system, and ameliorate, if possible, the condition of its victims. . . .

The causes of the supply have now to be examined; and first we may consider how far seduction operates in bringing women into the ranks of prostitution. It appears to be pretty generally admitted that uncontrollable sexual desires of her own play but a little part in inducing profligacy of the female. Strong passions, save in exceptional cases, at certain times, and in advanced stages of dissipation, as little disturb the economy of the human [female] as they do that of the brute female. . . .

That seduction in the proper meaning of the word can be charged with causing the unhappy condition of many of these unfortunate women is, I think, extremely doubtful; that numbers fall victims to the arts of professional and mercenary seducers is, I fear, equally true.

While visiting the Lock Hospital at Aldershot, the resident medical officer, Dr Barr, drew my attention to an interesting-looking girl, aged fifteen. As her case is one illustrating the fall from virtue of many another female, I may insert the story here, and can do no better than give it in Dr Barr's own words:

A few months since, E. P——, a pleasing-looking young girl, aged fifteen, was brought by the police to the examining room. I found it necessary, as she was painfully diseased, to detain her for treatment, and a few days since, being recovered, she was sent home to her parents. Her story is shortly, that for some months previously she had been nursemaid in a respectable family, but having quarrelled with her mistress, who was too exacting, and being very unhappy, she resolved to leave her situation. While on an errand one evening she met with a girl not much older than herself to whom she imparted her intention. This young person, who had lately been seduced by a soldier, and had heard a glowing account of Aldershot from him, told E. P—— of her intention to visit this place, and spoke of advantages they might both gain by travelling together. Unfortunately this girl's tale was too readily listened to, and that evening the subject of my narrative called on her parents, who are honest tradespeople in —— Street, Borough, and receiving from them some clothes, etc., without informing them of her intention, left London with her adviser on September 12 last.

Between London and this locality she was persuaded to yield to the solicitation of a man known by the girl with whom she travelled, but on arriving at the station and tiring of her companion, she separated from the latter, who remained in Aldershot. Afraid to return to her home she determined with imperfect ideas of distance to proceed to Yeovil, Somerset, where she believed some relative lived. The few shillings she possessed being soon spent she was forced to sell her bundle of clothes to procure food; and being by this time truly miserable, she resolved to go back to her friends, and retracing her steps again passed through a part of this district on her road to London. Without a penny remaining, weak for want of food, footsore and exhausted by travel, this poor young creature was accosted by the fellow alluded to above, who, quickly detecting her condition, commiserated her, and offered to supply her with food, clothing, and lodging if she would consent to meet a soldier or two who were friends of his. Alternate persuasion and threats overcame her resistance.

She was taken by her rascally protector to places where the soldiers congregate. A new and pretty face was sufficient attraction, and she became a toy for them during the evening; sleeping afterwards with 'Ginger', to whom, according to agreement, she handed the money received for her prostitution. This course lasted from the Friday of her arrival until the following Tuesday, her protector hiding her from the police in the daytime, but on the last-named day they took hold of her and brought her to me for examination. The girl's evidence having been heard, the parents were written to by Inspector Smith, and almost immediately the mother and sister came to see her.

Accustomed as I have been to witness meetings between those lost and their friends, and to listen to the heartrending details of sin and grief, I shall not easily forget the scene that occurred on this occasion. The mother, a well-conducted woman, told me that the family had been almost heartbroken by the sad event. As soon as it was known that the girl had left her situation without notice of her intention, they put an advertisement in *The Times*, and had numerous handbills printed and circulated, imploring her return. A whole month having passed without hearing anything of her, their misery can hardly be described, and to add to their unhappiness, the husband, a hard-working, industrious man, sustained a fracture of the leg, and was removed to a hospital. The poor mother, in the midst of her misfortune, fearing the worst results, whenever she heard of a body being found in the river or elsewhere, rushed to make inquiries, fully expecting to recognize her lost child in the inanimate form before her. Thus, until hearing from the police inspector, she was ignorant of the fate of her daughter during the period named. She finished by saying the girl had always been a good, engaging child at home; had, with the rest of the family, regularly attended Sunday school, and though poor, until this unfortunate occurrence, they had been a happy family. To make this sad story still more painful, and to add to the great affliction of this poor family, the girl is pregnant. The Association for the Protection of Women have taken up this case against the man referred to. A detective has been employed to search into the affair, and in the interests of humanity I trust he and similar scoundrels will receive their just punishment.

We have seen that many women stray from the paths of virtue, and ultimately swell the ranks of prostitution through being by their position peculiarly exposed to temptation. The women to whom this remark applies are chiefly actresses, milliners, shop girls, domestic servants, and women employed in factories or working in agricultural gangs. Of these many, no doubt, fall through vanity and idleness, love of dress, love of excitement, love of drink, but by far the larger proportion are driven to evil courses by cruel biting poverty. It is a shameful fact, but no less true, that the lowness of the wages paid to workwomen in various trades is a fruitful source of prostitution; unable to obtain by their labour the means of procuring the bare necessaries of life, they gain, by surrendering their bodies to evil uses, food to sustain and clothes to cover them. Many thousand young women in the metropolis are unable by drudgery that lasts from early morning till late into the night to earn more than from 3s. to 5s. weekly. Many have to eke out their living as best they may on a miserable pittance for less than the least of the sums abovementioned. What wonder if, urged on by want and toil, encouraged by evil advisers, and exposed to selfish tempters, a large proportion of these poor girls fall from the path of virtue? Is it not a greater wonder that any of them are found abiding in it? Instances innumerable might be adduced in support of this statement. I have said enough to acquaint the reader with the miserable condition of these

E

children of want; it is not my purpose to pain and horrify or to distract the attention from the main purpose of my book; those who desire a narrative of facts fully supporting this statement, I would refer to Mr Mayhew's work on *London Labour and [the] London Poor*. Misplaced love, then, inordinate vanity, and sheer destitution are the causes that lead to woman's fall and that help to fill the ranks of prostitution. But love should not lead to the forfeiture of self-respect. Vanity may be restrained; want may be relieved from other sources.

A still more frightful cause remains behind – more frightful because here the sinner has had no choice, so far as man can see, except to sin. Neither love nor vanity nor want have induced the surrender of virtue, for in this case virtue never existed, not even the negative form of virtue, the not-sinning state, the children of the very poor or very vile, what is their lot? It is a picture from which one recoils with horror, and the reality of which in this Christian country it is hard to believe. The cause to which I now allude is found in the promiscuous herding of the sexes (no other word is applicable through the want of sufficient house accommodation). I cannot better convey an adequate notion of the miserable dwellings of the very poor and the indecent mode of life resulting therefrom than by inserting the following extract from a letter written by Mr Mayhew to the *Morning Chronicle* some years since. If any doubt its accuracy, let them visit for themselves these wretched hovels, and see what barriers they form against decency and virtue. He says:

Let us consider, for a moment, the progress of a family amongst them. A man and woman intermarry, and take a cottage. In eight cases out of ten it is a cottage with but two rooms. For a time, so far as room at least is concerned, this answers their purpose; but they take it, not because it is at the time sufficiently spacious for them, but because they could not procure a more roomy dwelling, even did they desire it. In this they pass with tolerable comfort, considering their notions of what comfort is, the first period of married life. But, by-and-by they have children, and the family increases until, in the course of a few years, they number perhaps from eight to ten individuals. But all this time there has been no increase to their household accommodation. As at first, so to the very last, there is but the one sleeping room. As the family increases additional beds are crammed into this apartment, until at last it is so filled with them that there is scarcely room left to move between them. As already mentioned, I have known instances in which they had to crawl over each other to get to their beds. So long as the children are very young, the only evil connected with this is the physical one arising from crowding so many people together in what is generally a dingy, frequently a damp, and invariably an ill-ventilated apartment. But years steal on, and the family continue thus bedded together. Some of its members may yet be in their infancy, but other of both sexes have crossed the line of puberty. But there they are, still together in the same room – the father and mother, the sons and the daughters – young men, young women, and children. Cousins, too, of both sexes, are often thrown together into the same room, and not unfrequently into the same bed. I have also known of cases in which uncles slept in the same room with their grown-up nieces, and newly-married couples occupied the same chamber with those long married, and with those marriageable but unmarried.

A case also came to my notice – already alluded to in connexion with another branch of the subject – in which two sisters, who were married on the same day, occupied adjoining rooms, in the same hut, with nothing but a thin board partition, which did not reach the ceiling, between the two rooms, and a door in the partition which only partly filled up the doorway. For years back, in these same two rooms, have slept twelve people, of both sexes and all ages. Sometimes, when there is but one room, a praiseworthy effort is made for the conservation of decency. But the hanging up of a piece of tattered cloth between the beds – which is generally all that is done in this respect, and even that but seldom – is but a poor set-off to the fact that a family, which, in common decency, should, as regards sleeping accommodations, be separated at least into three divisions, occupy, night after night, but one and the same chamber. This is a frightful position for them to be in when an infectious or epidemic disease enters their abode. But this, important though it be, is the least important consideration connected with their circumstances. That which is most so is the effect produced by them upon their habits and morals. In the illicit intercourse to which such a position frequently gives rise, it is not always that the tie of blood is respected. Certain it is that, when the relationship is even but one degree removed from that of brother and sister, that tie is frequently overlooked. And when the circumstances do not lead to such horrible consequences, the mind, particularly of the female, is wholly divested of that sense of delicacy and shame which, so long as they are preserved, are the chief safeguards of her chastity. She therefore falls an early and an easy prey to the temptations which beset her beyond the immediate circle of her family. People in the other spheres of life are but little aware of the extent to which this precocious demoralization of the female amongst the lower orders in the country has proceeded.

But how could it be otherwise? The philanthropist may exert himself in their behalf, the moralist may inculcate even the worldly advantages of a better course of life, and the minister of religion may warn them of the eternal penalties which they are incurring; but there is an instructor constantly at work more potent than them all, an instructor in mischief, of which they must get rid ere they make any real progress in their laudable efforts – and that is, *the single bedchamber in the two-roomed cottage.*

Bad as are these pauper dens, nurseries of vice more fearful still abound in our Christian capital. In the former some effort after decency may be made, but in the latter, not only is there no such effort, but the smallest remnant of modesty is scouted and trampled down as an insult and reproach. I allude to the low lodging-houses which afford to the homeless poor a refuge still more cruel than the pitiless streets from which they fly. In these detestable haunts of vice men, women, and children are received indiscriminately, and pass the night huddled together, without distinction of age or sex, not merely in one common room, but often one common bed; even if privacy is desired, it is impossible of attainment; no accommodation is made for decency, and the practices of the inmates are on a par with the accommodation. It is fearful to contemplate human beings so utterly abandoned, reduced below the level of the brute creation. By constant practice, vice has become a second nature; with such associates, children of tender years soon become old in vice. This is no fancy sketch, or highly-coloured picture. In this manner thousands pass from childhood to youth, from youth to age, with every good feeling trampled out and every evil instinct cherished and matured; trained to no useful art, and yet dependent for a living on their own exertions, what wonder if all the males are thieves and all the females prostitutes. The crowding together of the sexes, and consequent indecency, is not entirely confined to the large towns.

My readers may recollect the effect produced by the letter of a brickmaker's daughter, when published in *The Times* for February 24, 1858. I subjoin portions of it bearing on the present subject:

My parents did not give me any education; they did not instil into my mind virtuous precepts nor set me a good example. All my experiences in early life were gleaned among associates who knew nothing of the laws of God but by dim tradition and faint report, and whose chiefest triumphs of wisdom consisted in picking their way through the paths of destitution in which they were cast by cunning evasion or in open defiance of the laws of man.

I do not think of my parents (long in their graves) with any such compunctions as your correspondent describes. They gave me in their lifetime, according to their means and knowledge, and as they had probably received from their parents, shelter and protection, mixed with curses and caresses. I received all as a matter of course, and, knowing nothing better, was content in that kind of contentedness which springs from insensibility; I returned their affection in like kind as they gave it to me. As long as they lived I looked up to them as my parents. I assisted them in their poverty, and made them comfortable. They looked on me and I on them with pride, for I was proud to be able to minister to their wants; and as for shame, although they knew perfectly well the means by which I obtained money, I do assure you, Sir, that by them, as by myself, my success was regarded as the reward of a proper ambition, and was a source of real pleasure and gratification.

Let me tell you something of my parents. My father's most profitable occupation was brickmaking. When not employed at this, he did anything he could get to do. My mother worked with him in the brickfield, and so did I and a progeny of brothers and sisters; for, somehow or other, although my parents occupied a very unimportant space in the world, it pleased God to make them fruitful. We all slept in the same room. There were few privacies, few family secrets in our house.

Father and mother both loved drink. In the household expenses, had accounts been kept, gin and beer would have been the heaviest items. We, the children, were indulged occasionally with a drop, but my honoured parents reserved to themselves the exclusive privilege of getting drunk, 'and they were the same as their parents had been'. I give you a chapter of the history of common life which may be stereotyped as the history of generation upon generation.

We knew not anything of religion. Sometimes when a neighbour died we went to the burial, and thus got within a few steps of the church. If a grand funeral chanced to fall in our way we went to see that, too – the fine black horses and nodding plumes – as we went to see the soldiers when we could for a lark. No parson ever came near us. The place where we lived was too dirty for nicely-shod gentlemen. 'The Publicans and Sinners' of our circumscribed but thickly-populated locality had no 'friend' among them.

Our neighbourhood furnished many subjects to the treadmill, the hulks, and the colonies, and some to the gallows. We lived with the fear of these things, and not with the fear of God before our eyes.

I was a very pretty child, and had a sweet voice; of course I used to sing. Most London boys and girls of the lower classes sing. 'My face is my fortune, kind Sir, she said,' was the ditty on which I bestowed most pains, and my father and mother would wink knowingly as I sang it. The latter would also tell me how pretty she was when young, and how she sang, and what a fool she had been, and how well she might have done had she been wise.

Frequently we had quite a stir in our colony. Some young lady who had quitted the paternal restraints or, perhaps, been started off, none knew whither or how, to seek her fortune, would reappear among us with a profusion of ribands, fine clothes, and lots of cash. Visiting the neighbours, treating indiscriminately, was the order of the day on such occasions, without any more definite information of the means by which the dazzling transformation had been effected than could be conveyed by knowing winks and the words 'luck' and 'friends'. Then she would disappear and leave us in our dirt, penury, and obscurity. You cannot conceive, Sir, how our young ambition was stirred by these visitations.

Now commences an important era in my life. I was a fine, robust, healthy girl, 13 years of age. I had larked with the boys of my own age. I had huddled with them, boys and girls together, all night long in our common haunts. I had seen much and heard abundantly of the mysteries of the sexes. To me such things had been matters of common sight and common talk. For some time I had trembled and coquetted on the verge of a strong curiosity, and a natural desire, and without a particle of affection, scarce a partiality, I lost – what? not my virtue, for I never had any. That which is commonly, but untruly called virtue, I gave away. You reverend Mr Philanthropist – what call you virtue?

Is it not the principle, the essence, which keeps watch and ward over the conduct, over the substance, the materiality? No such principle ever kept watch and ward over me, and I repeat that I never lost that which I never had – my virtue.

According to my own ideas at the time I only extended my rightful enjoyments. Opportunity was not long wanting to put my newly-acquired knowledge to profitable use. In the commencement of my fifteenth year one of our be-ribanded visitors took me off, and introduced me to the great world, and thus commenced my career as what you better classes call a prostitute. I cannot say that I felt any other shame than the bashfulness of a noviciate introduced to strange society. Remarkable for good looks, and no less so for good temper, I gained money, dressed gaily, and soon agreeably astonished my parents and old neighbours by making a descent upon them.

Passing over the vicissitudes of my course, alternating between reckless gaity and extreme destitution, I improved myself greatly; and at the age of 18 was living partly under the protection of one who thought he discovered that I had talent, and some good qualities as well as beauty, who treated me more kindly and considerately than I had ever before been treated, and thus drew from me something like a feeling of regard, but not sufficiently strong to lift me to that sense of my position which the so-called virtuous and respectable members of society seem to entertain. Under the protection of this gentleman, and encouraged by him, I commenced the work of my education; that portion of education which is comprised in some knowledge of my own language and the ordinary accomplishments of my sex; – moral science, as I believe it is called, has always been an enigma to me, and is so to this day. I suppose it is because I am one of those who, as Rousseau says, are 'born to be prostitutes'. Common honesty I believe in rigidly. I have always paid my debts, and, though I say it, have always been charitable to my fellow-creatures. I have not neglected my duty to my family. I supported my parents while they lived, and buried them decently when they died. I paid a celebrated lawyer heavily for defending unsuccessfully my eldest brother, who had the folly to be caught in the commission of a robbery. I forgave him the offence against the law in the theft, and the offence against discretion in being caught. This cost me some effort, for I always abhorred stealing. I apprenticed my younger brother to a good trade, and helped him into a little business. Drink frustrated my efforts in his behalf. Through the influence of a very influential gentleman, a very particular *friend* of mine, he is now a well-conducted member of the police. My sisters, whose early life was in all respects the counterpart of my own, I brought out, and started in the world. The elder of the two is kept by a nobleman, the next by an officer in the army; the third has not yet come to years of discretion, and is 'having her fling' before she settles down.

The extreme youth of the junior portion of the 'street-walkers' is a remarkable feature of London prostitution, and has been the subject of much comment by foreign travellers who have published their impressions of social London. Certain quarters of the town are positively infested by juvenile offenders, whose effrontery is more intolerably disgusting than that of their elder sisters. It is true, these young things spring from the lowest dregs of the population; and, from what I can learn of their habits, their seduction – if seduction it can be called – has been effected, with their own consent, by boys no older than themselves, and is an all but natural consequence of promiscuous herding, that mainspring of corruption among our lower orders. That such as these are generally the victims of panders and old *débauchées* is as untrue as many of the wretched fallacies set about by some who write fictions about social matters in the guise of facts; but whatever the prime cause of their appearance in the streets as prostitutes, it is none the less strange and sad – none the less worth amending – that the London poor should furnish, and London immorality should maintain, so many of these half-fledged nurselings, who take to prostitution, as do their brothers of the same age to thieving and other evil courses, for a bare subsistence.

Although a large number of women fall victims as above, it cannot be denied that others early evince a natural indisposition to do work when they might obtain it, and may thus be said to court admission into the ranks of prostitution. That idleness and vanity are almost inevitable bequests from parent to child, is proved by the fact that the children of the numerous diseased prostitutes, consigned by the police to the St Lazare Hospital in Paris, notwithstanding all the religious teachings of the Sisters of Charity and the excellent secular education given them within the walls of that institution, where they are received as old as seven or eight years, almost invariably become prostitutes. The foundlings, or deserted children, oftentimes illegitimate, who crowd our workhouses, are in like manner a very fruitful source for the recruitment of the metropolitan *pavé*.

With the absolute neglect of children by parents, and the interminable scheming of lustful men, I may end the roll of causes which have operated in this direction since the dawn of civilization, and, singly or combined, will so continue, I presume, to operate for all time.

7

REGULATION OF PROSTITUTION

I CANNOT venture to hope that the sexual passion will in our time cease to operate or diminish very materially. I have no idea that the preventives of prostitution hereafter suggested, will, if adopted at all, operate otherwise than tardily and incompletely. It becomes us, then, to consider what curatives or palliatives are at our disposal. Having already attempted to depict, not extravagantly, the present external aspect of the vice, and the interest of society in its being well ordered, I will now consider the possibility of our regulating it by law, or mitigating its attendant evils.

We may here at once discard from our calculation the class of females who live in a state of concubinage. Their ill effect upon society, so long as they remain in that category, is moral, not physical. They do not, or according to my theory previously illustrated, they very rarely descend into the grade of public supply, but are, even on the Continent, and still more in this country, utterly beyond the reach of medical or public police supervision. The depravation of public health and the national power are more traceable to the young clandestine prostitute, and the promiscuous class who practise from year's end to year's end, for five, ten, fifteen, or twenty years of their lives in a chronic or intermittent state of unsoundness. The hardened common prostitute when overtaken by disease, pursues her trade as a general rule, uninterruptedly, spreading contagion among men in spite of her own pain, that she may live and avoid debt, until positively obliged to lay up for medical treatment, in lodgings or in a hospital. It is from her class that society may be prepared for – if not expect – contempt of and danger to public order and decency; and over it the police of foreign countries have established the partial control already described.

In Chapter 4 I considered the working of the Contagious Diseases Act at Aldershot and other places, and approved the objects that it has in view, and the means adopted under its provisions, for lessening the evil results of the system against which it is directed. I showed that whatever opinion might be held by myself, or others, as to the advisability of interference on behalf of the general mass of the community, it was plainly the duty of the legislature to afford relief and help to those who through its action, rather than their own vice, are exposed to contaminating and hurtful influences. We have seen that its results, from a sanitary point of view, have proved most beneficial, and I earnestly advocate that every place in which there are barracks for soldiers, and all seaport towns, should be brought within its healing influence. The further question now arises whether its benefits should be confined to the present objects of its care, or be extended to the civil population.

On the propriety of adopting this latter course there is naturally great divergence of opinion, and some confusion of ideas. It is of the first importance that all who take part in the discussion should clearly understand their opponents' ideas and their own. It is happily a question far removed by its nature from the arena of party warfare, and the highest and most sacred interests of society demand imperatively that it shall not be made for party purposes the sport of rival politicians. It is, however, peculiarly susceptible to the influences of *prejudice and ignorance*, and we who desire by our labours to benefit the human race, must jealously guard against allowing our opinions to be warped by these twin enemies of truth. Some approach this question with selfish views, and desire to obtain by legal enactments immunity from danger in the gratification of base desires, while others, regarding prostitution as the safety-valve of society, wish to preserve, at the expense of others, their own wives and daughters from contamination. For such cold-blooded reasoners I have only the most unmitigated abhorrence and contempt; their maladies and pain deserve no sympathy, and as for their wives and daughters, I can only join in the indignant remonstrance, 'who are they that they should be considered while others are left to perish?' Surely, in the eye of their Maker, the noblest lady in the land is no more precious than the poorest outcast, and the fair fame of the one is too dearly purchased if the price be the other's virtue. For the credit of humanity, I trust that such views are not widely held, and that few desire the perpetuation of this loathsome system. A life of prostitution is a life of sin, replete with evils both for those who follow it as a calling and for those who reap advantage from their shame. As such it can receive from Christian men neither countenance nor toleration. This negative statement is too cold; it is their plain duty to do all in their power to discourage and repress it.

I have already shown that the evil is in its nature highly complex, its causes are various, and of divers degrees of endurance and intensity; of some of them, it may be fairly said that they are ineradicable and coextensive with human nature. So long as society has existed, its hideous counterfeit has been seen side by side and intermingled with it; and so long as society endures we may safely predict that it also will remain a foul reproach to Christianity and civilization, a puzzle to philanthropists, statesmen, and divines. Two propositions must be clearly kept in view: the one, that it is a sinful system, highly displeasing to Almighty God, and offensive to all right-minded men; the other, that until the world is purified from sin its extinction cannot be expected; and as a corollary to this last, I may add that it is an unextinguishable source of serious mischief.

The question then arises, what is to be done with this system, at once injurious, imperishable, utterly sinful and abominable? There are, as we have seen, two methods of dealing with it, diametrically opposed to each other, in vogue in the civilized world. The one is adopted on the Continent, and the other is adopted in England, and also in the United States. The former is the licensing, the latter the voluntary. They are of course based on entirely opposite principles. The LICENSING SYSTEM takes for its basis the indestructible nature of the evil and the terrible mischiefs which arise both socially and physically from its uncontrolled and misdirected energy; it is argued that it is better to recognize what we cannot prevent, and to regulate it rather than leave it to itself, and since we cannot suppress, to define the conditions subject to which it shall exist. The VOLUNTARY SYSTEM is based on the proposition that prostitution exists in defiance of the laws of God, that the only recognition which the State may lawfully take of sin is to suppress it, and that if this is inexpedient or impossible, the only alternative is to leave it to itself to find its own level and its own remedy – to remit to the individual conscience the abstaining from or partaking in the sin, and to private philanthropy the alleviation of its attendant evils. The State, in fact, ignores its existence, taking cognizance only of it indirectly, when gross acts of public indecency and disorder enforce attention and demand repression. It is objected to the licensing system, that it is in fact licensing sin, and that permitting indulgence under certain restrictions is in truth lending the sanction of the law to evil practices; it is also objected that it is practically useless, as the large majority of prostitutes contrive to evade its provisions. This is, however, not so much an objection against the system as an observation upon the method of carrying it out, and even if it be taken as an objection against the system, it seems to be one of little weight, because the facts are clear that several thousand women are thereby rendered physically harmless, that is to say, not merely a small, but a very large amount of good is done. Surely the refusal to reap a considerable benefit because we cannot reap all the benefit we desire is not wise. We should always bear in mind that half a loaf is better than no bread. It may, however, be said that the argument is not quite fairly represented, and that what is really meant is that the benefits derived from the licensing system are insignificant when compared with the evils introduced by it. The licensing system legalizes vice by distinctly permitting it under certain given conditions, the result of which is to lend to prostitution the appearance, at least, of a lawful calling, and to diminish sensibly both in men and women the sense of shame. Such a lowering of the public morals is too dear a price to pay for partial security to the public health. Another argument is, that it is degrading to the woman to be forced to publicly admit herself a harlot, and that English prostitutes would never submit to any law compelling them to do so.

It is a somewhat curious style of arguing, to tell us in one breath that the system is bad, because it takes away from the shame naturally attaching to the life of a prostitute, and in the next that it is bad because it increases her degradation, and takes away, if submitted to, the last remnant of self-respect – that it is bad because it accords a certain recognized position to prostitution, and exalts it almost to the dignity of a profession, thereby diminishing or destroying the sense of shame at their calling felt, or supposed to be felt, by prostitutes, and making them consider themselves, at the worst, 'martyrs to sensuality', to use the words of a celebrated *fille de joie*, and at the same time bad because it adds to the woman's sense of degradation, by compelling her to enrol herself publicly in the ranks of a shameful calling. If the calling have ceased, by the operation of the law, to be a shameful one, there is no degradation in admitting publicly connexion with it; if there is degradation in making this announcement, then has the trade not ceased to be shameful. These propositions cannot both be true at once; objectors to the licensing system must choose between them, and probably if they take their stand upon the first, their position will prove impregnable.

It is further objected that the licensing system encourages the trade of the brothel-keeper, and that to increase the security against disease is to diminish the sanction against indulgence, and thereby directly promote vice; it is asserted, in support of this view, that the tone of morals at Aldershot has visibly deteriorated since, and in consequence of, the passing of the Contagious Act; this last assertion must be strictly proved before its truth can be admitted, or its value, as an argument, acknowledged. And of the virtue, which is only preserved from fear of pain, we may fairly observe that it is a sufficiently cheap and poor possession, hardly worth protecting . . .

Whatever may be the failings of the licensing system, the demerits of the voluntary seem not inconsiderable. This latter is a systematic refusal to admit certain facts and their consequences, whose existence no sane person would attempt to dispute, or even casual spectators fail to observe, a perverse determination to ignore the presence of a vast mass of evil, because the best way to deal with it, is difficult to discover; the result is that disease carries on its ravages unchecked, private charity being unequal to the task of combating an enemy so gigantic. Our streets are a standing disgrace, the police being unable, with the limited authority intrusted to them, to cope with the disorderly characters that throng them. The great mischief of the licensing system is, that it tends to blunt the moral sense; of the voluntary system, that it leaves an evil state of things unchecked; this latter, out of regard for private liberty, neglects the public good, the former, for the supposed benefit of the State, remits to and confirms in a life of degradation individual members of the nation. It is difficult to choose between two evils, but happily for us the question is asked, and should be fairly answered, is there not some middle path that may be safely followed? Cannot prostitution be checked and regulated without being licensed? The Contagious Diseases Act exhibits an attempt to steer between these two extremes. It may be that some of its provisions are open to criticism; but critics should not confound two systems utterly different in principle. Though to a certain extent analogous in their working, both involve the recognition of prostitution – both enforce the examination and detection, if diseased, of the prostitute. The one, however, licenses the plying of a shameful trade on certain conditions fixed by law – in fact, legalizes the system. The other proceeds on the theory that it is useless to deny or ignore the fact that prostitution exists, and that worse evils even than those which now oppress us might be apprehended from any attempts to repress it, and that to strive to put it down is therefore worse than useless; but at the same time, that it is a thing to be kept within certain bounds, and subjected to certain restraints and surveillance. By the Contagious Act we virtually say to the women, 'You cannot be prevented from following this sad career which you have chosen; we cannot force you to abstain from vice; but we can and will take care that your shameful lives shall no longer work injury to the health of others, or outrage public decency.' Some assailants of the Contagious Act seem to confound it with the licensing system, and adduce arguments against it, to which, though the latter is plainly obnoxious, it most certainly is not. I hope that I have said sufficient to show how entirely different the two methods really are. We must not confound recognition with licence; to license prostitution is to license sin, and in a measure to countenance it. Recognition is not licence, and has neither the appearance nor the effect of encouraging vice. We are told that it is unchristian to recognize and make provision concerning fornication. Is fornication, it may well be asked, a greater sin than adultery? Yet the law recognizes and provides for this. Can it be said by the establishment of a Divorce Court to encourage adultery? Does it, in providing for the separation of faithless spouses, countenance their unchastity? Does it legalize adultery? Such a contention is absurd; it merely recognizes the fact that some people are untrue to their marriage vows, and provides the relief demanded by their unhappy cases. In the same way the law, in recognizing and legislating concerning prostitution and its attendant evils, neither encourages, countenances, or legalizes it.

Recognition is the first step necessary to be made by those who would oppose any effectual barrier to the advance of prostitution. In vain do we build lock hospitals and penitentiaries to heal or reform those who by accident, as it were, have fallen into sin and reaped its bitter fruits. Wilfully assuming, in spite of well-known facts, that the unfortunates relieved by our charity are mere waifs and strays of society, instead of being integral parts of a widespread system, poor stragglers that have fallen into a ditch, and been bruised and soiled in their fall, whom it is sufficient to extricate if possible, leaving the ditch untouched, in the hope, perhaps, that it will in time be cleansed by some accidental stream of purity, or choked up, it may be, by its own filth; whereas these saved ones are mere units out of thousands who have fallen into a deep and widespreading morass, which claims fresh victims yearly, and yearly encroaches on the honest soil around, who may for a brief space struggle to regain their footing when first made alive to the full horror of their position, but who, unseen or unpitied and uncared for by the passers-by, soon cease to struggle, and, helpless and hopeless, fall little by little, till they finally sink overwhelmed in the black depths of the treacherous swamp. To what good general end do we rescue a few of these poor sufferers from time to time, as chance may favour, leaving the multitudes to perish, and, worst and most fatal folly, leaving the morass untouched, to extend as it pleases, and engulph all it can? To leave an open stinking ditch unclosed is bad enough – to leave the morass untouched is fatal. To know of its presence and its power, to feel it close to us and round about us, and to think that we can free ourselves from its fatal influence by gazing on fertile plains around, or admiring the secure ground on which we ourselves are standing, is to act no better than the stupid ostrich, who hopes to elude her pursuers by shutting her eyes to their approach. To take no steps to control its power, while we build far from its brink a few poor refuge houses, insufficient to contain one thousandth part of the fallen ones, into which they may struggle if they can, unhelped by us – nay, rather pushed farther in – by way of dealing sufficiently with the mischief, is simply to reproduce Dame Partington's experiment with the Atlantic Ocean. What if the folly pleases and gratifies us? then let us at least remember that its result is the ruin of human souls – the pollution of the social fabric. What we have to do is to close the approaches to this deadly swamp – to drain it, and to fill it up, and at the same time to disinfect its foul malaria streams, and prevent them from overflowing into purer soil – to diminish its power for mischief – to stop aggregations to it – to withstand its extension. To do all this, we must take its measure, probe its depths, and accurately experience and understand its nature. We must look at it ourselves, and call the attention of others to it; we must discard euphemisms, and call it by its true name; we must prescribe the method of treatment, appoint its limits, and subject it to rule. What is this but recognition? The

public are, I am happy to believe, at length awakening to a consciousness of the truth of this position, and the principle has received
by the passing of the Contagious Diseases Act the sanction of the
legislature, so that accomplished facts have to a certain extent closed
the mouths of religious objectors.

It is still, however, unhappily true that the difficulties the philanthropist and surgeon have to meet in dealing with this subject are
raised mainly on its moral and religious side. Those who would ameliorate the physical condition of prostitutes on behalf of society are
at once met by the objection – 'Disease is a punishment for sin';
'syphilis, the penalty paid by society for indulgence in fornication';
and many worthy persons are so deeply impressed with these convictions, as to say, 'We will have none of your sanitary or preventive
measures, in this respect at least.' And again, 'The present chances
of contracting disease is the strongest means of deterring men from
being unchaste. This risk is the most potent barrier against vice.
Remove it, and you put a premium on fornication, discourage
matrimony, and upset society.'

It must be my endeavour to show the real value of this kind of objection, and further, to advance views which I trust may not be
deemed incompatible with Christianity and good morals. I admit,
without hesitation, that the fear of contracting contagious diseases
operates with many a gentleman of education and refinement as a
deterrent from fornication, and that such afflictions, involving, as
they in general do, both bodily suffering and financial loss, exert a
major force upon the unlimited recurrence to debauchery of the
poor, coarse, incontinent rake; I allow that, without this pressure,
men's sexual passion is so strong, and the training to continence
has been so neglected, that a life of sensual indulgence would, in the
present state of society, be more a rule than an exception; and I know
that it exercises some little influence even when religion is unheeded,
especially among the bulk of the better educated youth, whose minds
are so little made up upon the sinfulness of fornication, that I believe
the fear of suffering on earth operates more as a curb upon its
licentious practice than the more remote contingency of punishment
hereafter.

But, conceding this certain amount of deterrent power to the
liability to disease, we shall look in vain for proof that it has had any
effect towards extirpating the calling of the harlot, or the traffic in

female virtue, which has of late years forced itself upon the attention of our legislature. For every thousand upon whom it operates there are ten thousand thoughtless, passionate, habitually licentious men, on whom all lessons are thrown away, and as many defiant scoffers at religion and morality, who will point out some grey-haired offender, permitted by Providence to 'go on still in the way of his wickedness', for every 'frightful example' that can be adduced on the other side.

As I am writing this, a very remarkable case, showing how little deterring a cause is syphilis from vice, occurred to me.

In the early part of my practice, a gentleman of position was brought to me by his medical attendant suffering from severe affection of the bones of the nose, following several attacks of syphilis. Under our care the patient recovered, but lately the disease has returned, and just now this patient is under my care, not only on account of a piece of bone that I have removed from the nose, but he has come to me with two new chancres, contracted recently when taking his holiday. I may mention that my patient has a wife and family. He confided to me that his sexual passions were very strong, and when he takes wine, as he freely and habitually does, he is very liable to expose himself in spite of the danger, the importance of which he is fully aware of.

The following characteristics of prostitution are worthy of observation: First, that it must be co-existent with human society, a social plague that cannot be got rid of. That women who have abandoned themselves to this course of life are, nevertheless, susceptible of good influences, and capable of improvement and reformation; and, moreover, eventually return for the most part to a more regular mode of life. That many enter upon this life owing to evil rearing, or driven by want. The first seems to point to the necessity of regulation, the second to amelioration, the third to prevention. I propose in this and the succeeding chapters to consider the subject under these three heads; and first regulation, as, having arrived at the conclusion that prostitution must always exist, it seems reasonable to consider how far it admits of regulation, before turning our attention to plans that may be adopted for amelioration or prevention. Prostitution cannot be put down, though its extent may be diminished and its attendant evils mitigated. It seems to admit of regulation in three particulars – viz., the health of the women, their places of resort, their appearance and demeanour in the streets. I have already sufficiently shown the great mischief that arises to the community from the presence in our midst of vast numbers of diseased prostitutes. We have seen that the voluntary system encourages the existence and spread of infectious disorders, evils which are, on the Continent, sought to be obviated by the licensing system, which however is open to the serious objection that it is in fact licensing sin, that it makes the State an accomplice in wickedness, and results, as might be expected, in hardening the consciences of men and completing the degradation and ruin of the prostitute. Any change to it, therefore, from the voluntary system, notwithstanding all the mischiefs to which the latter exposes us, is out of the question. We have also seen that a measure has been recently adopted in parts of this empire for dealing with disease fairly obnoxious to none of the defects chargeable upon the licensing system, although it has been attacked with more zeal than wisdom on similar grounds.

It is not my purpose to merely force opinions of my own upon the reader. I have set before him the evils to which we are exposed, and the methods of dealing with prostitution adopted in this and other countries. I am deeply conscious of the difficulties that beset our efforts to bring about a better state of things, and that it becomes a reformer to be tentative rather than dogmatic in his speech. I will therefore, instead of attempting to form any system of my own, call the attention of the reader to the evidence of Captain Harris, one of the Commissioners of Police, before the Committee of the House of Lords in June, 1868, as to the advisability of extending to the civil population the provisions of the Contagious Diseases Act. I cannot do better than give the evidence *in extenso*, with the addition of a few remarks of my own upon it:

Can you give us any ideas as to how far it is practicable to extend the Act to London? – I consider it very feasible. Knowing the object of the committee, I have prepared a paper upon the subject of this inquiry, which, if you will allow me, I will read:

'The prevention of contagious diseases being an object of primary importance, I beg to suggest that the operation of the Contagious Diseases Act, 1866, might, with advantage, be extended to the civil population of the metropolis. I would recommend that a special department of police be formed, similar to the common lodging-house branch, now in operation. That this department should consist of two divisions, administrative and active. That the administrative should be 1 chief inspector, 1 registering inspector, 1 serjeant clerk; and that the active should be 4 visiting inspectors, 20 visiting serjeants.' I name a very small staff in the first instance, because it is easier to extend than to reduce the number. 'That this department be entrusted, (1) With the surveillance of houses of ill-fame, to enforce cleanliness and good order; (2) To maintain decency in the streets with regard to public morality; (3) To suppress the sale of indecent prints, photographs, etc.; (4) Repress, as far as possible, clandestine prostitution; (5) Apprehend procuresses; (6) Apprehend persons who procure abortion; (7) Search for women who fail to attend medical inspections. That to this department be entrusted the registry of prostitutes within the district. That no prostitute be registered unless, (1) There be proof of former offences; (2) Public notoriety, such as attendance at places of public resort, or where prostitutes assemble, or other form of conclusive evidence. That each registered woman be required to carry a card, on which shall be entered, (1) Name; (2) Address; (3) Date of last medical inspection. The following regulations should be printed on the back of this card: (1) To show card when demanded by officers of police specially employed in this department; (2) To present themselves every fortnight for medical inspection; (3) Not to stop or form groups in the public thoroughfares.

'I recommend that there should be a compulsory periodical medical examination of all females known to be prostitutes, and of all unmarried soldiers and sailors; more particularly previous to the former going on or returning from furlough; or when the latter are on board a harbour ship. As the early treatment of the disease is indispensable, examination, when persons are supposed to be diseased only, is insufficient; besides, irregular examinations are objected to by the females themselves. The absence of regular and frequent examinations allows the disease to be communicated before discovered. It is necessary that ample hospital accommodation be provided; that the patients may be detained in hospital as often as found diseased, and as long as they continue so; and that when discharged from hospital, the discharge ticket be handed to the police to prevent its improper use. Under the present system there is a constant influx of diseased women into towns where the Act is in operation, showing the necessity of applying preventive measures to all places. Should the Act become general, it would be necessary to provide hospital accommodation in all unions of parishes.' (I presume half a dozen beds, in country districts, would be sufficient.) 'Some difficulty might be experienced at first from the want of sufficient hospital accommodation; I would recommend the establishment of hospital ships under the charge of naval surgeons; these vessels might be dispensed with as the disease lessened. I recommend that there should be a weekly medical examination of all women living in brothels; and that all drunken prostitutes charged before a magistrate should be medically examined before being discharged. It is found, where the Act has been in operation, that the more serious forms of disease are of rare occurrence; that the social condition of the prostitutes has been raised; that their homes and habits are improved, and that they are more cleanly in their persons. No objections would be raised on the part of these unfortunate women to the surveillance of the police of this special department; the common lodging-house serjeants are much respected by the lower orders, and considered in the light of friends; and I feel assured that these unfortunate women would at all times look to the police for protection.'

You have used the phrase, to suppress 'clandestine prostitution': how would you propose to do that? – The examination that these women would be subjected to, would cause a great many to abstain from prostitution.

It has been proved that that has been the result of the Act, in places where the Act has been carried out? – Yes, it has.

Is that the only mode by which you would suppress clandestine prostitution? – The fact of women being subjected to medical examination would, in a great measure, prevent their entering into that course of life.

Then the simple carrying out of the extension of the Act, as it now stands, would effect that object? – I think so.

Then you would simply propose a special police, to carry out the Act as it now stands, with the addition, as I understood your paper, of Lord Campbell's Act, against immoral prints? – The police carry out the provisions of Lord Campbell's Act, at the present moment; but I would suggest that directions be given to this special branch of police to carry out the provisions of this Act.

Then, as far as I can make out, you would make no change in the Act, except extending it, and supplying the police to work it? – Yes, and making the medical examination compulsory.

It is compulsory already, is it not? – Yes; but from a want of sufficient hospital accommodation, the provisions of the Act are not enforced. I strongly advocate the registering of women, because I think that you cannot reach the whole of them unless they are registered.

That is the mode by which you would get hold of them, namely, by registering? – Yes.

You think that the Act, as it now stands, requiring an information before a magistrate, is insufficient for getting hold of all the common prostitutes? – Yes. I think that there might be other clauses introduced into the Act.

To what effect? – I think that, if the Act were properly carried out by the police, houses of ill-fame might come under the control of the police. At the present moment the police do not interfere with these houses; for instance, in Portsmouth they have no control over them.

But as I read the Act, if a woman has got the disease in a brothel, the brothel-keeper is liable to punishment? – Yes, if he does not give information of the existence of the disease. (*The Act is handed to the Witness.*) He is liable to a penalty, I see, for harbouring. 'If any person, being the owner or occupier of any house, room, or place within the limits of any place to which this Act applies, or being a manager or assistant in the management thereof, having reasonable cause to believe any woman to be a common prostitute, and to be affected with a contagious disease, induces or suffers her to resort to or be in that house, room, or place for the purpose of prostitution, he shall be guilty of an offence.'

Earl De Grey:[38] I think your attention has been drawn to clauses 15 and 16 of the present Act? – Yes.

Do you not hold that under the 16th clause there is the power in justices to order the periodical inspection of any woman who may be represented to them, upon the oath of a superintendent of police, as being a common prostitute? – Yes.

Whether she be diseased or not at the time when that statement is made to the magistrate? – Yes.

Therefore, those clauses give the power in that respect which you think it would be desirable to extend? – Yes.

But I understood you to say that power was not universally acted upon even in the districts to which the Act now applies, in consequence of insufficient hospital accommodation? – Yes, from the want of sufficient hospital accommodation, the provisions of the Act are not enforced.

Then the defect in that respect arises not from the fault of the Act, but from the want of hospital accommodation? – Yes.

You spoke of the keeping of a register of these women. The police at present exercise a certain control over common prostitutes; do they keep any register now of those people in London? – No, they do not.

But your suggestion that a register of these women should be kept, would not, I suppose, involve the granting to them of any licence as prostitutes? – No; certainly not.

Would you approve of a licensing system? – No; I do not think that it would be desirable.

You think that it would be repugnant to the general feeling of the country, I suppose? – I do.

What distinction do you draw between a licence of that kind, and the certificate which you suggested should be given? – That certificate would be simply a card to be produced to the special branch of police (provided one was established), to enable them to see where the woman resided, and whether she had undergone the periodical medical examination.

That card, then, would simply be to show that she had complied with the provisions of the Act? – Yes.

At present, I think, in all the places in which the Act is now in force, whether at dockyards or at military stations, the carrying it out is entirely entrusted to the metropolitan police? – It is.

If the Act were to be extended to other districts of the country, not containing naval or military establishments, it might be difficult to extend the power of the metropolitan police there, might it not? – I think that great difficulty would be found in that respect.

Do you think that the ordinary county constabulary could carry out the Act? – I think that the county constabulary might, but I should be sorry to entrust it to the hands of the borough police, except in such towns as Liverpool, Manchester, Bristol, etc.

In the larger towns, you think, where there is an efficient police, the Act might be carried out by the local constabularies? – Yes.

But that would be difficult in the case of smaller towns? – Yes.

Earl of Devon:[39] You select picked men for this purpose now, do you not? – Yes.

Do you select men of a certain age? – No.

Are they married? – Two-thirds of our men are married; so that, in all probability, married men would be selected to carry out the Act.

Viscount Sidmouth:[40] In places like Devonport and Portsmouth, I suppose the police are tolerably well acquainted with the women of the town? – Yes, they are well known to them.

Are there occasions of a great influx of fresh women? – Yes.

These would be immediately known to the police, I suppose? – Yes.

Would it not be easy for the police to have authority to see that in any case of an influx of fresh women, they should be subjected to examination, because the police would know the parties to pitch upon, would they not? – Yes, they would know the parties; but at the present moment, with the very limited hospital accommodation at our command, it is useless to have them examined, as you cannot send them into hospital, even if found to be diseased.

What I mean is this, that it would be possible for the police to have power to compel these women to be examined, and not to exercise their vocation until they had passed this examination, and that, in the case of their doing so, they should be liable to some penalty? – That would be quite possible; but I do not think that power exists at the present moment.

Will you state whether you have known many cases where penalties have been inflicted under the 36th clause, for it seems to me that there would be some difficulty in getting a conviction for a person harbouring a prostitute, and 'having reasonable cause' to suspect that she has the disease? – I do not think that there has been a single conviction under that clause.

Or a conviction for keeping brothels? – No, there has been no conviction under this Act for keeping a brothel.

The conviction can only take place where the keeper of that house has 'reasonable cause to believe any woman to be a common prostitute, and to be affected with a contagious disease'? – Yes; that is to say, for carrying on her calling, she being in a diseased state.

But you have not known cases of conviction at present? – No, I do not think that there has been a single conviction.

Earl De Grey: You suggest now that any prostitute brought before a magistrate for being drunk and disorderly should be inspected before being discharged; and I suppose that you would add, should be sent to the hospital if found to be diseased? – Yes.

Is the number of prostitutes who appear before magistrates on charges of that kind a large number? – There must be a very large number in the course of the year.

Would they form a large proportion of women of that character? – Yes, of the very low prostitutes round about Wapping and Shadwell, and in that neighbourhood.

Lord Penrhyn:[41] You spoke of insufficiency of hospital accommodation just now: have you ever known any instances at Portsmouth or Aldershot of women being taken into the workhouse when suffering from the disease, in consequence of the deficiency of hospital accommodation? – No, I do not myself know any case of the kind.

You are aware that there is a clause in the Poor Law Amendment Act enabling the guardians to retain any person in the workhouse suffering under contagious diseases? – Yes.

You do not know whether it is acted upon or not? – No.

Earl of Devon: Do you know cases where the guardians have refused admission into workhouses to women suffering under this disease? – No, I do not know of any such case.

Viscount Templetown:[42] Is the attention of the policemen selected for this particular duty strictly confined to that, or do they exercise all the other functions that belong to the police? – I think that they exercise their ordinary functions; if they saw any case of felony committed, or assault demanding their interference, they would interfere.

You are, I suppose, aware of what occurs among the police at Chatham and Sheerness, and Devonport and elsewhere? – Yes.

Have you ever heard of any violence being shown towards them on the part of these women? – No.

The police perform their duties with ease? – Yes; there is no difficulty whatever.

Lord Penrhyn: Do not you think that it would be difficult to frame any Act by which a line could be drawn as to women above the class of common prostitutes? – I do not myself think that there is the slightest difficulty whatever in that.

In what way would you propose that it should be drawn; I am speaking of the class of woman who is above solicitation in the street, who comes above the class of common prostitutes, and yet is known to carry on this intercourse with men; where would you draw the line? – Speaking of London, I should propose that any woman who goes to places of public resort, and is known to go with different men, although not a common street-walker, should be served with a notice to register.

Is there anything that you could take notice of beyond that fact of a woman going to public places and going with men from those public places; you could not draw the line, so as to inquire into people's character, to know whether they had connexion with men or not, could you? – It would be soon known to the police; every woman has a place of resort, and I think the police could find out any woman's history in London, if they chose.

Do not you think that it would be difficult to draw the line in an Act? – I do not consider that necessary; I think that every common prostitute should be registered, and a day named for medical examination. It would be desirable to classify, as far as possible, the women for this purpose, a certain day in the week being set apart upon which medical examinations would be made by payment; this would enable the better class of women to classify themselves, and would partly defray the expenses of putting the Act in operation. Great discretion, however, is necessary in carrying out an Act such as that contemplated.

Viscount Templetown: Do you know whether the police employed in carrying out this Act obtain their information from the prostitutes themselves, or from the men? – I think they obtain information from the men; but I do not consider that you can in every case rely upon it; it is difficult for a man to say that he got the disease from any particular woman.

Do you think it would be difficult, from the information they possess, for policemen to find out from prostitutes whether any prostitute among them is diseased? – I think they might readily find it out from the women; the women would tell upon one another.

Do you see any reason why it should not be an indictable offence when a woman, knowing herself to be diseased, gives disease to a man? – No, I see no reason why it should not be made so.*

We learn from the above evidence of Captain Harris, that he considers the idea of extending the Act to London very feasible. He has from his position ample opportunity of judging, and his experience and ability lend great weight to his opinion. . . . There is a twofold disadvantage in placing some districts under surveillance and restriction, from which adjoining districts are free. In the one case, prostitutes plying their trade in the former are

* [*Report from the Select Committee of the House of Lords on the Contagious Diseases Act, 1866* (1868), qq. 742–800.]

enabled to baffle the vigilance of the police, to defy the law, and spread disease, by living in the adjoining districts, thus adding greatly to the immorality of these places. This is very noticeable in the country districts around Oxford and Cambridge, more especially the latter. For the purposes of discipline at the Universities, large powers are entrusted to certain officers called proctors, part of whose duty is to prevent any intercourse between undergraduates and women of the town, the latter being liable to arrest and imprisonment if caught *flagrante delicto*; the result is that the majority of the women take up their headquarters in the adjoining villages and towns outside the jurisdiction of the proctors, thus introducing an immoral element into places which would otherwise be comparatively free from taint. The other disadvantage is, that diseased women flock in from the free districts, to those under supervision, to obtain for themselves the benefits of medical inspection and hospital nursing, thus pressing unfairly on the resources of the district and the time of the medical staff. If all places were made subject to the same supervision this double evil would be avoided.

With regard to the machinery to be employed, it is only natural that Captain Harris should incline to entrust the police with the carrying out of the Act, and they are no doubt the proper persons to perform the subordinate duties; the public, however, are naturally, and it seems to me very justly, jealous of vesting administrative power in the police, who are, and ought to be, nothing more than servants of the executive; and even if this were not so, it is at least a question whether so difficult and responsible a duty could be safely remitted to the unaided discretion of police inspectors: they are, as a rule, undoubtedly worthy men, but it is no disparagement to them to say that the person responsible for the action taken should be of superior position and education; and I would suggest that the police should act under the orders of medical officers, it being of the greatest importance to guard against tyrannical and indiscreet behaviour in the performance of the difficult duties created by the Act.

It does not seem to me that the surveillance of any houses of ill-fame, except accommodation houses, should be considered part of the duty of the police, as for reasons that I shall give in another place, I am inclined to think that, with this exception, such places should be altogether repressed. It is difficult to know what offences the assistant-commissioner requires that a woman should be guilty of to justify her registration as a prostitute, and it is to be regretted that his evidence is not more explicit on this point, as the question what conduct is to expose a woman to police surveillance is one of no small difficulty.

I subjoin here the presumptions of prostitution required on the Continent, before placing a woman upon the registry; not that I wish it to be supposed that I advocate their adoption *in toto*, or that I consider that they afford the only or the best criterion to judge by, but because it seems to me that I shall best assist the reader to form an opinion on this difficult point – what course of conduct is to render a woman liable to be placed on the police registry as a common prostitute – by placing before him all the facts within my knowledge that appear to bear upon it. The points, then, from which presumption of clandestine prostitution are deduced on the Continent, are the following:

1. When a girl is arrested in any public place or public road, giving herself up to acts of debauchery with a man who declares he does not know her, and will not bail her.

In this case the offence of clandestine prostitution is complicated with the offence of outraging public feeling and modesty, and often that of vagrancy.

2. When a girl is arrested introducing into her house a man whom she has met in the public streets, or place of public resort, and who makes the same declaration as the above.

3. When a girl is arrested in a furnished house or inn, shut up with a man who makes the same declaration as the above.

4. When in a short period the police have met the same girl in the streets, or public places, with different men, although each of them may have declared themselves to be her sweetheart or her protector.

5. When a girl has been arrested in a house of accommodation, or when the police see her entering or leaving a house of this description.

6. Associating with well-known prostitutes, or the mistresses of houses of ill-fame, is considered presumptive evidence of clandestine prostitution.

In any of these cases, and on a written report signed by two policemen, the girl is summoned before the *Bureau des Mœurs*, by letter; and if she refuses to come she may be arrested and brought by force before the chief of the *Bureau*. She may then be examined as regards her family, her antecedents, her business, etc., and a letter is written to the mayor of the town in which she says she was born; if subsequently it is found that she has renounced work, and has no other means of subsistence than prostitution, if found affected with venereal disease, and it is in vain to hope that she will return to an honest way of living – permission is asked from the mayor or the prefect, to inscribe her on the register of public prostitutes.*

I regret to observe that Captain Harris is inclined to recommend that a card should be given to the prostitutes when registered; this has too much the appearance of the health ticket of the foreign *inscrite*, and if not intended to be used in the same way is certainly very adaptable to the purpose. The only reason for giving this card seems to be to facilitate identification by the police; a little additional trouble on their part seems a good substitute for it. Captain Harris agrees that the licensing system is undesirable. It is imperative to avoid not only the reality, but also the appearance of it. It will be seen that more hospital accommodation is necessary for the extension of the Act, and even for the proper working of it in its present state, as the question of greater hospital accommodation requires attention, whether any change such as here suggested is made in the law or not. I shall deal with this subject hereafter in the chapter on amelioration, to whose pages it seems more properly to belong.

One serious objection presents itself at once to the mind of an Englishman, when measures of surveillance are suggested to him; it is sufficiently well founded, to require to be fairly encountered and fully answered, or else frankly admitted to be fatal. The objection is, that such measures are invasions of private liberty, and therefore intolerable in the land which boasts itself to be the peculiar home of freedom. The slave who sets foot on English soil is free, and here the fugitive from tyranny finds refuge and shelter. We may go where we like, do what we like, say what we like, be what we like, so long only as we obey the laws. And these laws are framed with the object of securing to the individual the largest amount of liberty consistent with public welfare. This personal liberty, the birthright and heritage of every Englishman, purchased by our fathers' blood, and

* Jeannel, *De la prostitution* (1868), 227–9.

secured by the wisdom and labours of centuries, is a noble possession to be preserved by us undiminished, and by us transmitted to the after-time unshorn of any of its fair proportions. This is not merely a sacred duty, but an instinct in our nature, so that when any change is proposed that seems to encroach upon a right so precious, we may expect it to be regarded with suspicion, and encountered by resistance, and doubly so when the objects of its attack are mean, defenceless, and despised. Moreover, this English liberty includes the right to sin as much as we please, so long only as we do not thereby commit any offence cognizable at law, against the property or person of our fellow subjects. We may gamble, drink, and whore; the first must be done to a certain extent in private; the second must not cause public commotion; but the last may be done without any restriction whatever.

Every man is free to seduce a woman, take his neighbour's wife, or keep a mistress, without rendering himself obnoxious to the penal law. He may be a sabbath-breaker, atheist, or teacher of sedition, and yet incur no punishment. In like manner it is undeniably lawful for a woman to abandon herself for money if she chooses. This right of sinning, however, infinite though it at first sight appears, is subject to certain restrictions, and even actions, in themselves innocent, may fall under the scourge of the law if indulged in under circumstances prejudicial to the public safety. For instance, there is no harm in stone throwing *per se*, but if little boys, or others of a playful disposition, throw stones at railway trains, or in places of public resort, they by so doing render themselves liable to punishment; and in the same way it is unlawful to let off fireworks in the streets, or to ride full gallop in Rotten Row. Again, there is no harm in selling goods at a shop – on the contrary, it is a very praiseworthy means of earning daily bread; but the fishmonger who sells stale fish, the butcher who sells tainted meat, and the tradesman who uses false weights, are liable to punishment. And this, notwithstanding that it would be quite possible to do substantial justice between the dishonest trader and his customer, by leaving the latter to recover damages for the injury done to him in a civil action; *caveat emptor* is a sound maxim, the buyer has his own folly to thank if he is taken in. And again, there may be no buyer at all, and therefore no one is actually taken in. The mere fact of endeavouring to trade with the bad fish, or meat, or the false weights, is an offence against the law.

It will no doubt be objected that there is no parallel whatever between the case of a dishonest trader and a diseased prostitute – that the former is pursuing a lawful calling, and that people come to his shop with an honest object, and therefore that it is only right that they should be protected by the law; while to the latter it is impossible that a man should go with an honest purpose, and therefore the law rightly extends protection in the one case, which in the other it withholds. There is, no doubt, much force in this observation; it must not, however, be carried too far; and it must be remembered that the gist of these offences is, in the one case, doing acts that may prove injurious to the public health, in the other attempting to obtain money under false pretences; and the fact that any injury is actually done on the one hand, or any money actually obtained on the other, is not material to constitute the offence. The question remains, does the immorality of the transaction through which the injury must come in the case of the prostitute, place the infliction of the injury, or the attempt to inflict it, beyond the cognizance of the law? I think not, and will produce a case in point.

Gambling is, in the eye of the law, immoral, and its public practice prohibited, so much so, that not only are public gaming tables suppressed, but even wagering on horse races is prohibited in the streets, and in public-houses. If any man, therefore, loses his money gambling, he has only himself to thank for his folly; and had he not engaged in an immoral transaction, he would have been secure against the loss. So that it was through his own evil deed that the loss befell him; and yet if money is unfairly won at games of chance, the cheat is liable to punishment for obtaining money under false pretences. The reason is obvious; gambling, although a wrong thing, and a pursuit which, therefore, the law will not encourage, is very widely indulged in. It is quite impossible for the law to put it down; it is plain that, in spite of any enactment that might be passed against it, men would still yield to the indulgence, and therefore the law punishes those who play unfairly. No man would willingly play with a cheat, neither would any man in possession of his senses knowingly go with a diseased woman. The cases are analogous; why should not the law insist in both on fair play, that what is actually given should correspond with what is professed to be given; and why should the law punish the individual taking advantage of human weakness in one case, and not in another?

We have, then, in the law against unfair gaming the principle admitted that punishment may be meted out to those who in immoral transactions, which the law takes no other cognizance of, act in a manner injurious to others. Although the victims of the unfair play are themselves engaged in an immoral pursuit, and have thus exposed themselves, through their own fault, to evil machinations, those who take an unfair advantage of them are punished. But here again we find a difference; the law does not interfere until the crime has been committed. The law attempts no surveillance of gamblers, but this is because the law will not attempt impossibilities, and it would be impossible for the police to exercise any surveillance over persons unknown to them. It may be objected that in the proposed registration of prostitutes, a whole class will be placed under certain disabilities, quite irrespectively of any given individuals comprising that class, being in such a state as in the particular case to make inspection necessary. To this it may, I think, be fairly answered that when persons commit themselves to a course of life which may, and in the majority of cases does, actually render them dangerous to the public health, the law may reasonably interfere with their liberty, so far as to insure that as little evil as possible may result to the State from their immoral practices; in fact, we may go a step further, and say that it is only right that this should be done, and that personal liberty and personal rights must be in all cases subservient to the public welfare. Compulsory vaccination is a case in point: here the law interferes plainly and directly with the liberty of the subject; parents may dislike to have their children vaccinated, and it may be that in nine cases out of ten the precaution is superfluous; still there is a certain danger that must be guarded against, and private inclination and opinion must yield to the exigencies of public safety.

The laws for the suppression of betting-houses establish another principle, which is, that persons who will persist in doing an immoral thing, must not do it in such a manner as to place temptation in the way of the thoughtless and ignorant, and, by a parity of reasoning, the law may insist that if women will pursue the shameful trade of prostitution, they must do so in such a manner as not to place temptation in the way of those who might otherwise abstain from immorality. The laws protecting minors from dealing with their property or binding themselves by contracts, and married women from being sued for debt, or dealing with their property, except under certain conditions, furnish a further instance of protection being afforded by the State to persons in an otherwise defenceless condition. The young and inexperienced are peculiarly liable to yield to the temptations of harlots and to suffer the evils incident thereto: for their protection, therefore, if for no other reason, the law may rightly place restrictions upon prostitutes. Further than this, large numbers of the lower classes are, as we have seen, almost forced by circumstances into a vicious mode of life. Surely it is not too much to ask the law to protect them so far as possible from the evils attending the accident of birth.

We have thus far argued the case, merely from the point of view of protecting others; may we not add a plea on behalf of these unhappy women themselves? Is it not a worthy object to force these wretched creatures to pay some attention to cleanliness and health, to bring healing and elevating influences within their reach, to raise them, if not to virtue, at least from the lowest depths of degradation, to bring to them relief from suffering and help in distress? For the sake of these wretched women, no less than on behalf of the rest of the community, this act of mercy should, it seems to me, be passed. One other instance of interference for the public good with private liberty must not be unnoticed: the Habitual Criminals' Bill which, while these sheets are passing through the press, has received the sanction of the legislature, strongly asserts this principle. Under its provisions, persons may be committed to prison, not for overt acts of crime brought home to them by regular legal process, but because they are known to be leading lawless and predatory lives. No principle is more clear or more jealously asserted than that every man shall be presumed to be innocent until proved to be guilty; but here the burden of proof is shifted, and guilt is presumed until innocence can be shown. This Bill, and especially, perhaps, the clause relating to receivers of stolen goods, is a far more arbitrary enactment than the measure that we are considering. The laws restraining nuisances and compelling unwholesome and noisome trades to be carried on in such places and in such a manner as to interfere as little as possible with the health and convenience of the community are clearly restrictions for the public good upon private liberty, as also are the laws permitting the compulsory surrender of private property for the public advantage. I think that I have now said enough to show that the principles involved in this measure are already sanctioned and acted upon in numerous instances. A paternal government, as it is called, is intolerable to English instincts, and will ever, I hope, remain impossible in this country. People must be left to a great extent to reap the bitter consequences of sin and folly, but the principle lying at the very root of the existence of society is, that for the common good and for the advantages obtainable by this means only, each member of the State must be content to be deprived of the power to do exactly as he pleases – that is, must surrender for the sake of social order a portion of his freedom. So much for the arguments that may be adduced against the proposed legislation on the ground of interfering with the liberty of the subject. But after all, what is this liberty? It is not liberty, but wanton license. It is not freedom, but lawless indulgence. . . .

The law is cognizant of the existence of prostitution. It is known that thousands gain their bread by lives of infamy; the evils incident to and arising from their calling, also, are well known. May it not be urged with at least equal truth that the law that permits without restraining is in reality an accomplice, and chargeable with the evils which it refuses to remedy. 'Am I my brother's keeper?' was the excuse for himself, offered by the first murderer, and is virtually said by all who see suffering and wrong, and pass by on the other side. Let us beware lest in endeavouring to avoid a sin, we do not fall into a greater. The suffering shame and ruin ascend from the pitiless streets and haunts of misery to the gates of heaven, and cry there for vengeance, not only on those who wring from broken hearts their guilty pleasures, but also on those who, wrapping close around them the cloak of self-righteousness, and shutting up their bowels of compassion from the sorrow that they needs must see, refuse to make even an effort to avert it, or to raise the arm, which if stretched forth, might save.

After all, the question resolves itself to one of common sense. Does the Contagious Diseases Act, so far as tried, work well? I appeal with confidence to results. *Si monumentum quaeris circumspice.*

* * *

From discussing the advantages derivable from a systematic supervision of prostitutes, we pass on to the question how far it is possible to control their appearance and deportment in public. In dealing with this part of my subject, I propose first to consider what steps, if any, should be taken with regard to the various places to which they resort. These naturally divide themselves into two distinct heads: the first comprises the casinos, music-halls, and public gardens, such as Cremorne; the second, the class of places known as night-houses.

I must here, again, remind the reader that prostitution must always exist, that it cannot be suppressed by law, and that no measures taken against it will be wise and beneficial which do not recognize this fact. It cannot be denied that the existence of places where prostitutes congregate is an enormous evil. The attempt to suppress them all would, however, be as impolitic and quixotic as the attempt to suppress prostitution itself. All that we can do, is to render the public haunts of prostitutes as little injurious to the public morals as their nature admits of. Although this is undoubtedly true, it does not follow that every place is to be tolerated. It will be seen that the two divisions above referred to are very different in character, the one existing for other purposes besides that of affording facilities to the practice of prostitution, the other for this purpose alone. I think that we may lay down and act upon the following principle, that all places of which the only use is to enable women to meet with customers should be rigorously repressed, but that such places as exist for other objects, such as music or dancing, although it may be true of them that they are supported mainly by base women and their associates, must be tolerated. The first division, therefore, must be permitted to continue as at present.* With regard to the second, this again divides itself into the night-house proper, such as Kate Hamilton's, Rose Young's, Coney's,[43] etc., etc., where refreshments are supplied without a licence, and after the regular hours, and from which the police are so far as possible excluded, and the supper-rooms and cafés in and about the Haymarket from which the police are not excluded, and in which refreshments are not supplied without a licence; it would be as unreasonable to deprive a prostitute of a place for obtaining refreshment as to close against her all places of amusement; these latter, therefore, must be left unclosed, at all events for the present. The case of night-houses, however, is very different; they exist only for the purposes of vice, and

---

* I have had so good an exponent of my views in the following article, that I reproduce it: [see Appendix B, pp. 221–3].

should be put down with the strong hand. We have already seen . . . how difficult it is for the police to suppress these places in the present state of the law. I submit that it would be well to deal with them in precisely the same way as by the Habitual Criminals' Bill the persons obnoxious to its provisions may be dealt with; there is no question as to their character, the only difficulty being, to obtain such evidence of it as shall amount to legal proof and justify conviction. It seems to me that if the principle of the Habitual Criminals' Bill were adopted in their case, and the burden of proof shifted from the police to the ostensible proprietor, their suppression would be easily obtained.

From the night-house to the house of ill-fame the transition is easy. This latter class comprises, as we have seen, two distinct species of brothel: the brothel proper, or dress-house, where women are kept by the proprietor, and farmed for his benefit; and the accommodation house, where in return for a moderate payment the convenience of temporary shelter is afforded to chance companions. The first of these houses should, in my opinion, be utterly suppressed. I postpone, however, to the chapter on prevention, the discussion of this question. The second must, I think, be tolerated, and for the same reason that prostitution must be tolerated because their suppression is either impossible or attended with worse results than the mischiefs which they occasion. They are in fact rather the result of evil than the cause. True it is that in France they are viewed with more disfavour than the *maisons de filles*, but that is because the French system makes no efforts for the amelioration of the prostitute, but recognizes prostitution as a necessary evil, and those who follow it as a calling, as persons forming a certain defined class whom it is necessary to render amenable in the greatest possible degree to regulation; it therefore directs all its efforts to producing centralization; this process is assisted by the *maisons de filles* with their confined inhabitants, and retarded by the *maisons de passe* with their floating occupants. In England we recognize prostitution as a necessary evil in the same sense only as we recognize poverty, crime, and disease as necessary evils. The object of those who advocate regulation in England is not to create a class bound down by hard and fast limits, whose life and development are blighted and ruined, for the supposed advantage of the State. We want no 'martyrs to sensuality'. We admit the fact that prostitution must exist, and admitting it, and feeling its power for evil, we deprecate the policy of ignoring it, and demand that limits be fixed which it must not pass, and laws laid down for it that it must obey. We therefore suggest that those who are known to lead this life of shame, and to have no other means of subsistence than those afforded by prostitution, should be registered; and as the only way of checking the fatal evils arising to the community from their mode of life, that those persons whose names are found in the register should be compelled to submit to inspection. We know that the class must exist; we know the dangers to which by its existence we are exposed; we desire to limit those dangers, and to deprive the class so far as possible of the power of inflicting physical injuries.

But we desire more than this, we desire to ameliorate the condition of the individuals comprising that class, and to lessen their numbers. We see that the life of prostitution is in the majority of cases temporary only; we desire not to make it permanent. We see that prostitutes, . . . as a rule, return to the ranks of honest people and become absorbed in honest society. We wish therefore to ameliorate their condition, to elevate their habits, of thought and mode of life, so that their return may be assisted and accelerated, and that as little as may be of degradation may be absorbed in their absorption. The method, whatever it may be, by which our object can be best achieved, is evidently something very different from centralization. The motive, therefore, that makes the *maison de passe* in France peculiarly obnoxious to the law does not exist in England.

One other principle I may allude to here, which should be firmly held by all advocates of regulation, and should accompany the one that I have just stated, which is, that prostitution must so far as possible be kept a thing apart and by itself. Society must, so far as possible, be secured against its contaminating presence. We desire to give all possible access of good and helping influences to the prostitute, and to draw her back from her life of sin, but we must be careful in doing this not to give prostitution access to society. Fornication must not come to be regarded here as a *naughty* thing which everybody does.

I may now repeat and examine the proposition that houses of accommodation must be tolerated because their suppression is either impossible or attended with worse results than the mischiefs which they occasion. The main objections to them are the following:

they afford facilities for the illicit intercourse of the sexes; they keep in existence a class of people directly interested in the extension of prostitution; it will be more difficult for the police to make complete registers, if places are tolerated to which women can take their customers, instead of having only their own houses to take them to. To the first objection I answer, that it proves too much. Prostitution being permitted to exist, houses in which prostitutes live must also be permitted; to these they can take their customers, and it seems to me to make little difference whether the rooms to which men can be taken are regularly rented by these women, or by other people; no greater mischief seems likely to arise (except that arising from the other objections that I have stated) to the woman, her customer, or the public, from the existence of houses of accommodation than from the existence of houses where prostitutes live. The second objection is more serious; it is no doubt most undesirable that any people should exist interested in the continuance and increase of prostitution, or that any persons should gain advantage or earn their livelihood from the sin of others. On this subject, however, we are endeavouring to attain, not the desirable but the possible; the only legislation for which we can hope, is a balance of evil.

Rigorous enactments against bawds and panders will enable us to prevent the keepers of houses of accommodation from turning them into dress-houses, or brothels proper, and from promoting the extension which they desire of an evil system. While, as to the third objection, though we must regret any circumstance that may render more difficult the arduous duties which will, under the proposed system of regulation, fall to the lot of the police, we feel bound to say that any objections of this sort are of a secondary nature only; that although they must, if possible, be obviated, when this cannot be done the difficulty must be cheerfully accepted and means found to meet it.

Having disposed of the objections that may be urged to the toleration of houses of accommodation, I may now consider the reasons that seem to render their repression impolitic, and these fortunately come within the range of experience. We find that since the law has been put in force against these houses their number has been sensibly reduced; on the other hand, hotels, restaurants, and coffee-houses have been to a large extent pressed into the service of prostitution; thus is introduced the very mischief against which we desire to guard, namely that of bringing prostitution and society *en rapport*, so to speak. However deplorable it may be that accommodation houses should exist, it is infinitely more undesirable that through their extinction every coffee-house should become a brothel, and that hotels and restaurants should be generally, and as a matter of course, used for immoral purposes. In addition to this, any law for the suppression of these houses can be easily evaded, and in their absence means will be surely found to meet in some more irregular and objectionable way the requirements of vicious people.* Legislation, then, on this point is at best useless, and should therefore be carefully avoided.

The regulation of prostitutes' appearance and behaviour in the streets is the only other topic to which allusion need be made in this chapter. The police have, as we have seen, . . . power to arrest, if necessary, persons guilty of indecent and disorderly conduct in the streets. It seems hardly possible to interdict the prostitute from the liberty of using the public thoroughfares, which she naturally enjoys in common with the rest of the community, and it is a question whether the right can be denied to any one person of civilly addressing any other. These natural rights, however, of using the streets and addressing the passers-by give rise to the evils of loitering and solicitation.

The condition of our streets – although a marked improvement seems to have been effected in the interval that has elapsed since the appearance of the first edition of this work – is still far from satisfactory, and it is worthy of consideration whether, notwithstanding the right to which I have above referred, some further improvement may not be made in this respect. Of pertinacious solicitation there appears to be little or none, unless, perhaps, occasionally late at night. Against solicitation every man has the remedy in his own hands; it is, no doubt, a nuisance to which he should not be exposed, but as the absence of rejoinder usually suffices to repress it, and in the rare cases in which it proves insufficient, an effectual appeal can always be made to a policeman, it seems better to leave things as they are, at all events for the present, than to run the risk of introducing by stringent enactments more serious evils. It is, moreover, a ques-

* This objection is not an imaginary one. I understand that a limited liability company has already been started for providing its members with the accommodation they desire; doubtless more will follow.

tion of detail, fit rather to be dealt with by the Police Commissioners than worthy to be made the subject of legislation. This last remark applies with equal force to the question as to the best means of dealing with the mischief of loitering. It is to be met by applying to it some recognized principle rather than by direct legislation. I must, however, point out that certain localities are far worse than others: the question may arise whether in such of these as may happen to be merely bye-streets, any measures should be taken for the prevention of loitering, but it seems to me that all the principal thoroughfares should be protected from this nuisance, and this could be accomplished by a little firmness and tact on the part of the police.*

Of one thing we must not lose sight, and that is, the necessity of giving no opportunity to the police of indulging in acts of petty tyranny. The majority of the force are, I believe, men of good temper and behaviour; but no one acquainted with the streets of London can be ignorant that the instances of bullying and over-bearing conduct towards unfortunate costermongers, applewomen, and others are far more frequent than could be wished.† The first thing necessary, therefore, is, that the police authorities shall tell off for the duty of preventing loitering, those men only on whom they can implicitly rely – men who will act up to their authority, but not exceed it, and who will perform their duties not only with firmness, but also with gentleness, moderation, and discretion. The next step is to give these men full instructions to prevent the obstruction of the thoroughfares. The duty is, no doubt, a somewhat difficult one, but the exercise of common sense will suffice in the majority of cases to prevent the commission of any grave

* I may mention the street connecting Leicester Square with the bottom of Regent Street as a thoroughfare infested with loitering prostitutes from whose presence it should be freed,[44] the Burlington Arcade as a place the policy of interfering with which is open to question.

† A case of very recent occurrence illustrates and justifies my anxiety that no unnecessary power may be entrusted to injudicious officers. A respectable married woman passing through a locality much infested by prostitutes, and ignorant of her way, asked a passer-by for direction; she was immediately pounced upon by an over-zealous constable, and, despite her explanations and the remonstrances of the man to whom she spoke, was summarily walked off to the police station. What satisfaction to her for so gross an outrage was the severe censure ultimately administered to the policeman?

errors. 'I have often,' the late Sir P. Laurie once observed, 'discharged unfortunate women against what appeared to be the reasoning of the police, that if a woman after having walked down Fleet Street dared to walk back again, she must be walked off to prison.'[45] And the worthy alderman was undoubtedly right. If some modern Dr Johnson should propose to walk down Fleet Street, and having walked down should propose to walk back again, and should give like effect to the last proposition as to the first, and should repeat the operation a hundred times in the course of the day, 'the active and intelligent officer' who should attempt to interfere with him would expose himself to the charge of being foolhardy and unreasonable. In the same way a cluster of the gentler sex round windows dedicated to the display of bonnets, robes, or jewelry should not be wantonly disturbed. If, in the place of the learned doctor on the one hand, and the fair cluster on the other, we find a portly harlot or a collection of vicious women, the same observations will hold good. The pavement is free to all: to use, however, not to abuse. The book-making fraternity are not allowed to pursue their avocations in the streets; why should greater indulgence be extended to prostitutes? The action taken against betting men perhaps supplies the rule of which we are in search; and it may be safe to lay down that, making allowance for the difference of pursuit, the police should, in those cases in which they would interfere with these latter, interfere also with prostitutes, who should certainly be prevented from turning their promenades into short beats, and making any leading thoroughfare their daily haunt.

The foregoing suggestions seem to me sufficient as regards the regulation of the streets in the daytime and evening. As the night advances, the number of disorderly characters present in the streets increases; this is especially the case in those nearest to the places of amusement frequented by prostitutes and their companions. We have seen that the neighbourhood of the Haymarket has acquired an evil notoriety, and I think it is clear that the state of things existing in this and similar localities should not be tolerated. Although I have admitted that the liberty of using the streets should not be denied to women merely on account of their being prostitutes, there would, I think, be no harshness or undue interference with the liberty of the subject, in requiring such persons to withdraw from them within half an hour after the time at which the Argyll Rooms and similar places of amusement are usually closed. Some such measure as this seems absolutely necessary to prevent the continuance of a grave scandal, and we must not forget that if we make the streets less disreputable, we shall in doing so diminish both the opportunity for and the temptation to impure indulgence.

8

AMELIORATION OF PROSTITUTION

THE amelioration of prostitution has a twofold operation. It should be directed to the healing and cure of prostitutes suffering from disease, and also to accomplishing their social and moral elevation. Up to a very recent period I had believed that this was the wish of all interested in the welfare of women in the United Kingdom. My readers may imagine with what deep regret I read in the last issued report (the 11th) of the Medical Officer of the Privy Council[46] his official enunciation of the startling doubt '*Whether the venereal diseases of the civil population are henceforth to be deemed matter of public concern*'....*

Mr Simon, while coinciding in the view '*that prostitutes having relations with soldiers in garrison towns should be supervised by government*', is disinclined to extend the benefit of the Contagious Diseases Act to the civil population. He says:

> Of the venereal diseases of the civil population, English sanitary law has not hitherto taken any special cognizance; and whether this neutral state of the law ought or ought not to be abandoned is a separate question, of far more intricacy than seems to be generally imagined, and which on all acounts certainly deserves most careful consideration.†

And after giving various reasons which, whatever their intrinsic value may be, are apparently satisfactory to his own mind, thus states the conclusion at which he has arrived:

> The broad result in my mind from the various above-stated considerations is, that at present I very decidedly refrain from recommending any change in that neutral position which English law has hitherto held in regard of the venereal diseases of the civil population. So far

---

* [*Eleventh Report of the Medical Officer of the Privy Council . . . 1868* (1869), 18. Acton's italics.]
† [*Ibid.* 11.]

as my present knowledge enables me to judge, I believe that any departure from that position could do little but embarrass and disappoint.*

Venereal diseases are, in principle, infections which a man contracts at his own option, and against which he cannot in any degree claim to be protected by action of others – the less so, of course, as his option is exercised in modes of life contrary to the common good; that thus, *prima facie*, the true policy of Government is to regard the prevention of venereal diseases as matter of exclusively private concern. *Caveat emptor!*†

And again . . . he remarks:

Whether the venereal diseases of the civil population are henceforth to be deemed matter of public concern, *whether the civil fornicant may reasonably look to constituted authorities to protect him in his commerce with prostitutes*, is the principle which I conceive to be at stake.‡

From the above, and many similar passages to be found in this report, it would seem that Mr Simon conceives the sole object, which people advocating the extension of the Contagious Diseases Act to the civil population have at heart, is to provide immunity from suffering for self-indulgent and vicious men. This narrow conception of the views entertained by others, and of the important issues really at stake, must tend to deprive this report of much of the weight that might otherwise attach to it.

I must moreover enter my most emphatic protest against the method adopted by Mr Simon, of stating the question. I feel sure that he would not willingly attribute to those from whom he differs motives which do not actuate them; nor do I believe that he would wilfully raise a false issue; he has, however, in stating the principle which he conceives to be at stake, fallen into the error of treating as identical two propositions widely different. To the first proposition, and to that alone, we must look for the principle; and for that I venture to solicit an affirmative answer; for the second, in common with Mr Simon, and all right-minded men, I demand an indignant negative. The fallacy of stating these two propositions as identical is so transparent, that I should not have noticed it here only that it

* [*Ibid.* 16.]
† [*Ibid.* 13.]
‡ [*Ibid.* 18. Acton's italics.]

affords a striking illustration of the deep-rooted prejudice with which this question is unhappily interwoven, which confuses the understanding and judgment of men undeniably upright in their intentions, and possessed of undoubted ability. The first proposition presents us with 'a . . . question', to quote Mr Simon's own words, 'of far more intricacy than seems to be generally imagined, and which on all accounts certainly deserves most careful consideration'.* The second proposition has, so far as I know, never been put forward by anyone, and is, in fact, nothing more than an inaccurate statement of one of the many considerations with which we have to deal in coming to our conclusion on the first; and the proposition put forward by Mr Simon may be fairly stated thus: 'Whether the venereal diseases of the civil population are henceforth to be deemed matter of public concern, seeing that one necessary result must be that the civil "fornicant" will in that case receive a certain amount of State protection in his commerce with prostitutes.' Mr Simon's second proposition is, in fact, an exaggerated statement of the principal objection to his first.

It is, perhaps, unfortunate that any steps taken to stay disease and to alleviate the many evils that are brought by prostitution upon the community must tend to make commune with prostitutes less hazardous; but the real question that we have to consider is whether, seeing the infinite mischief brought upon society by venereal diseases and the action of prostitution generally, such matters should not henceforth be deemed of public concern notwithstanding the comparative immunity from suffering thereby secured for men of loose habits of life. To make the path of sin less dangerous to the sinner is no wish of mine, but I hold that a course fraught with benefit to society and to thousands of miserable women should not be abandoned merely because it entails this consequence with the rest. Towards the conclusion of the article, Mr Simon again indulges in language, that conveys both an odious imputation on his opponents and an unfair statement of the question at issue between him and them. When he considers 'hospitals for . . . prostitutes . . . as elements in a machinery proposed to be constituted by law for giving an artificial security to promiscuous fornication'.†

* [*Ibid.* 11.]
† [*Ibid.* 20.]

Surely scientific vituperation cannot go further than this. Is this the language which one of Mr Simon's supporters and critics has called vigorous? I trust my readers will agree with me that at least it is not convincing, and to them I confidently appeal to decide for themselves between the objections brought by Mr Simon against 'State interference to provide for the disinfection of prostitutes',* and the reasons which I give in this book for the extension of the Contagious Diseases Act to the civil population.

★   ★   ★

OBJECTION NO. I. Mr Simon thinks there are 'swarms' of ratepayers who would object to see the prostitute

kept in hospital at their expense for weeks or months, not necessarily from the exigencies of severe illness of her own, but essentially that she might be made clean for hire, lest any of her users should catch disease from her; they would remember in contrast, that for themselves wonderfully little is done by authority to protect them against adulterations of food, or against false weights or measures; and they might regard it as a strange caprice of law which should oblige them to contribute to the cost of giving an artificial security to their neighbour's looseness of life.†

This objection assumes (among other things) that the 'swarms' of ratepayers are all virtuous, and would neither for themselves nor their relations, such as sons or nephews, rejoice that life's temptations were made less full of pain and peril; that, though so stern towards civil naughtiness, they do not object to the expense of relieving the immoral disasters of soldiers and sailors; that the prostitute would not be sent to hospital on account of her own severe illness; that she would be so sent 'to enable her to hire herself out by being made clean'.

Now this is really too bad, fathering as it does unworthy motives on those who desire to secure efficient hospital relief for the sick prostitute. The injustice of these two last assumptions is equalled only by the grotesque absurdity of the argument that the hospitals

* [Ibid. 10. This phrase occurs in Simon's section-heading, and is italicized by Acton.]
† [Ibid. 12.]

ought to be closed to prostitutes, because sufficient attention is not paid to preventing the adulteration of food and the use of false weights and measures. Can we not obtain, if necessary, legislation for the relief of both evils? To refuse to do one thing because something quite different requires to be done, can only be wise on the supposition that two wrongs make one right. But, after all our grumbling as taxpayers, we must bow to the voice of public opinion which, as someone has well said, does not depend upon the opinion of one individual, but flows from the combined judgment of the 200 able-thinking men who constitute the working majority of our constitution.

While on this point, however, I may deal with the different objections that may be urged against providing relief and assistance in their dire necessity to fallen women. It may be objected that the suggested provision for prostitutes during sickness will directly encourage immorality by making prostitution less hazardous, the risk of destitution ensuing on the contraction of disease being calculated to operate as a strong deterrent to persons meditating its adoption as a calling. This objection is plausible, but not, I think, well founded. Women do not as a matter of fact calculate chances before entering on a career of prostitution, or if they calculate at all, it is the calculation of the gambler who dwells only on expected gains, and dismisses from his mind, if ever indeed the unwelcome possibility should cross it, the anticipation of probable loss, or if he condescends to dwell for a moment on a contingency so remote, he trusts that the happy chapter of accidents will enable him in some unknown but yet expected way to tide over the season of disasters. The choice of prostitution as a means of living cannot in my opinion be conceived even in this limited sense to be a matter of calculation; it is usually referable to accident, necessity, or vicious inclination. Such an objection, moreover, would be equally applicable to any attempt at ministering relief by private charity, and this even the most rigid of disciplinarians, including Mr Simon himself . . . would hesitate to condemn.

It may be further objected (as it has been by Mr Simon) that such provision is an unfair tax upon the virtuous and well-conducted, compelling them to support the vicious and improvident, even against their will, and that such support, if given at all, should at least be given voluntarily. The plain answer seems to me to be this:

175

the voluntary system has been fairly tried, and has been found wanting. In spite of the efforts of private philanthropy, prostitution and its attendant disorders, social and physical, oppress us heavily, and, according to Mr Simon, at least double the number of hospitals at present established are necessary to enable us to deal efficiently with metropolitan diseases. It is time to check the evil. Diseased prostitutes can no longer be permitted to infest the streets and spread contagion and death at their good pleasure. They cannot be kept off the streets except by being placed in confinement, and curing their diseases seems to be the necessary accompaniment of restraining their liberty.

It is, however, further urged that vicious men ought not to be preserved from disease at the expense of the virtuous. If prostitution were an evanescent evil this objection would, I confess, have weight; but, seeing that its nature is what I have already described it to be, I reply that, striking the balance of evils, the fewest are attendant on a system of regulation and amelioration. No method of dealing with it that human ingenuity can devise can be an unmixed good, and we must only be content in this as in other things to take the rough with the smooth.

But beyond and above all utilitarian reasons, one motive for adopting the course that I am now suggesting stands forth pre-eminent, and it is one that I commend to the careful consideration of all Christian readers. It is this. I have already shown that numbers of women have no choice fairly before them, except to join the ranks of prostitution, through the neglect, or even worse fault of society, rather than through their own deliberate sin. Women who, if born under happier auspices, might have proved virtuous and faithful wives and mothers find themselves vicious and despicable outcasts. Shall we, the prosperous and respected, who indirectly permit or produce their fall, feel under no obligation to seek for and apply the remedy? I say that it is the plain duty of a Christian State to place within the reach of all its members, even the vilest and lowest, the means of obtaining health; also, that it is its duty to place within the reach of all, so far as possible, the means of amendment and reformation. From those who urge the hatred of sin as a Christian duty I claim the exercise of another Christian duty, the showing mercy.

★ ★ ★

OBJECTION NO. 2. Mr Simon, however, further objects that even if advisable, the system would entail so enormous an expense for hospital accommodation as to render its rejection necessary. He says:

> To give a notion of the quantity of hospital accommodation which would be requisite to satisfy this programme, I may observe, for instance, that London is conjectured to have some 18,000 women whose living is gained by prostitution; and that, according to one of the secretaries of the society, on any given number of prostitutes, always about one-third may be assumed to be diseased. If, instead of insisting on these colossal estimates, we take only half their total result, the plan would require for London alone the creation and maintenance of new hospital accommodation nearly equal to that which is now given by the twelve general hospitals of London for all bodily diseases put together: accommodation, namely, for 3,000 patients. The charge of maintaining (independently of the cost of constructing) such lazarets as the above would, probably, be at least £100,000 per annum: and their construction would probably represent a first cost little short of half a million of money: besides all which there would be the considerable annual charges for police arrangements and medical inspections. This for London alone! And the requirements of other large towns would probably be of like proportions.*

Mr Simon does not acquaint us, as I think he should, with the statistics and calculations by which he arrives at his estimate of the probable cost of dealing effectually with Metropolitan prostitution; the only figures that he gives he has himself taken from others; but these carry us a very short distance in the calculation – no further, indeed, than the starting point. Mr Simon cannot assume that out of the given number of 9,000 prostitutes there will, under a system of supervision, be a perpetually recurring quantity of 3,000 diseased women. Such an assumption would contradict the result of all our recent experience, and be simply ridiculous. But it is useless to speculate on the process adopted by Mr Simon; I am unable to form any hypothesis from the facts and figures known to me by which his calculation can be supported. If his conclusion is the result of mere guesswork, it would have been at least candid to say

* [*Ibid.* 11–12.]

so; if he is in possession of facts, figures, or other information not generally known to the profession, he should in justice to himself, the profession, and the public, produce them. . . .

OBJECTION NO. 3. The next objection, which, if proved, would have great weight with the authorities and the public, is the statement made by Mr Simon:

> On the other hand, as regards our power of preventing venereal diseases by such a superintendence of prostitution as is proposed, it is certain that no appreciable good would be got except with much organization, and at very large cost of money; and there are strong reasons for believing that the gain so purchased would, on analysis, be found to belong very predominantly to those kinds of venereal disease in which the community has little or no permanent interest.*

The real fact is, that it is *precisely these forms of disease in which society is most interested*, which have been most beneficially influenced by the system of inspection now in practice, and that it is on the slighter and less important forms that the least impression has been made. . . .

In the London Lock Hospital, as previously stated . . . Mr Lane reports that in 1867, 42 per cent and in 1868 only 35 per cent of the prostitutes admitted laboured under syphilis, thus showing that the working of the Contagious Diseases Act has very considerably diminished the syphilitic average.

OBJECTION NO. 4. Mr Simon doubts the success of the Continental system; he says:

> Then, as regards the preventability of venereal diseases, even the abstract question (abstract I mean from considerations of cost) is by no means an easy one. Especially we are in want of exact discriminative information as to the good which other countries have got from their sanitary superintendence of prostitution. I believe it to be the fact that, even under strict systems of police, prostitutes in very large proportions escape the intended supervision; and that in their evasive traffic so large a dissemination of venereal diseases may be kept up as to leave in net result very little apparent success to be boasted of.†

My reply to this objection is, that I do not propose to apply to

* [*Ibid.* 14.]
† [*Ibid.* 15.]

England the system in vogue on the Continent, but one apparently less obnoxious to the prostitute (that at present carried out in our garrison towns), and therefore likely to be in a far less degree the object of evasion.

No one can read the statistics . . . without being convinced that the system has had the effect of immensely diminishing the severity and frequency of disease in the several European capitals. In speculating as to the benefits derived, or derivable, from a system of supervision, it must be remembered that the good achieved by it will be great in proportion as the area made subject to it is extensive. . . .

OBJECTION NO. 5. Mr Simon appears to infer that the extension of the Contagious Diseases Act to the civil population would discourage early marriage by favouring fornication; for he says:

> I suppose it may be assumed that public policy is very decidedly in favour of marriage as against promiscuous fornication; that the latter, however powerless may be laws to prevent it, is at least an order of things which no State would willingly foster.*

And again:

> The only state of things which can be regarded as essentially antagonistic to prostitution is the system of early marriages: which, in this respect, commends itself equally on moral and physical grounds; for, in proportion as it is accepted, the promiscuous intercourse of the sexes ceases to excuse itself by circumstances, and the chances of venereal infection fall to the lowest level they can attain.†

I was not aware before, that Government considered marriage in this sense. I thought that in the present state of crowded civilization political economists had come to the conclusion that early marriage was an evil, and have always heard Ireland cited as an instance of its ill effects. . . .

In a medical point of view I have elsewhere shown that early marriages are followed by the worst consequences to the rising generation. Premature procreation is bad for the male, injurious to the female, and detrimental to the children . . . But whatever may be the intrinsic value of early marriages, whether from a political, social, or

* [*Ibid.* 12.]
† [*Ibid.* 19–20.]

medical point of view, the sufficient answer to this suggestion of Mr Simon's is, that it is impracticable. As reasonable was the demand of the King of Egypt for bricks without straw, or the proposal of the French Princess that the people should have recourse to pastry who, from the scarcity of flour, could get no bread, as this recommendation to men to take wives who have not wherewithal to support them. If the only state of things essentially antagonistic to prostitution is out of our reach, we must discover and apply some less transcendental remedy. At the same time, it remains open to Mr Simon to show, first, that early marriages will counteract prostitution; and secondly, that the Government can, and will, by an improved system of emigration, or otherwise, place them within the reach of prudent men.

OBJECTION NO. 6. Mr Simon doubts the moral results of Government superintendence on prostitution. That gentleman says:

Among arguments put forward to recommend a general superintendence of prostitution, there is one which seems to have gained for the proposal a considerable quantity of non-medical, particularly clerical, support. The report of the Association,[47] namely, alleges 'that a collateral but not unimportant result which inevitably follows the establishment of preventive measures is the improvement in the moral and social condition of the women'; and a memorial which was last year addressed to the then Lord President of the Council, by the President of the Royal College of Physicians and others, supported the view 'that of the unfortunate women who are subjected to these restrictive and sanitary measures, a comparatively large proportion have been reclaimed'. I believe it to be unquestionable that such women as have hitherto come under medical inspection have generally been influenced by it to become cleanlier in their persons, and that the brothels inspected by police are less apt than they were to be scenes of riotous disorder; changes, on which no doubt the users of those persons and places may congratulate themselves; but which cannot without extreme abuse of terms be described as of any moral significance. On the other hand, the last clause of the statement cannot fail to seem morally important to anyone who accepts it without reserve. I fear, however, that such hopes as it at first sight would seem to justify, as to possible moral results of a government superintendence of prostitution, would on any large scale show themselves essentially delusive; not perhaps as regards individual reclamations to be effected, even from brothels, by pure and kindly human contact, but as regards the statistics of prostitution, broadly and practically considered.*

Surely this is a rash assertion for Mr Simon to make, immediately after the publication of the report of the House of Commons for 1869, a report which, I cannot too often repeat, contains most valuable information. It says:

Although the Act has only been in operation two years and a half, and at some stations only seven months, strong testimony is borne to the benefits, both in a moral and sanitary point of view which have already resulted from it.†

The evidence I have adduced in the former edition of this book – that even when the English Government held a neutral position as regards prostitution, the prostitute had a tendency to withdraw herself from the paths of vice, and to settle down into a gradually regular life, till she became often a mother of a family – becomes of still more importance now that State interference interests itself on her behalf.

The partial Government garrison superintendence has . . . had a most beneficial influence, and there is every reason to believe that if steps continue to be taken for further extending the Contagious Diseases Act, we shall have a beneficial change in the moral and social condition of the class such as nothing else can effect. . . .

I verily believe that if I had not been convinced that a large number of the women who practise prostitution settle, and become valuable members of society, I should not have exerted myself as I have done to better their condition. To take advantage of and assist this tendency towards the marriage state, has been the object of much of what I have written. I have insisted over and over again in these pages that it is not my object to benefit the user of the prostitute, or, to again employ the language of Mr Simon, keep a prostitute 'in hospital . . . that she should be made clean for hire, lest any of her users should catch disease from her'.‡

* [*Ibid.* 18–19.]
† [*Report from the Select Committee on Contagious Diseases Act (1866)* (1869), p. iii.]
‡ [*Eleventh Report of the Medical Officer . . .*, 12.]

In combating the introduction of the Contagious Diseases Act into civil life, Mr Simon has entirely ignored this ultimate amalgamation of prostitutes with the population. If there are only 18,000 prostitutes in London, does it not become of the greatest importance that the State should first protect them, next cure them, and then assist an erring sister in forsaking what has become to her a vile occupation? . . .

Prostitution is a transitory state, through which an untold number of British women are ever on their passage. Until preventive measures . . . shall have been considerately adopted – and thereafter, too, if needful, for I am no nostrum-monger – it is the duty, and it should be the business of us all, in the interest of the commonwealth, to see these women through that state, so as to save harmless as much as may be of the bodies and souls of them. And the commonwealth's interest in it is this – that there is never a one among all of these whose partners in vice may not some time become the husbands of other women, and fathers of English children; never a one of them but may herself, when the shadow is past, become the wife of an Englishman and the mother of his offspring; that multitudes are mothers before they become prostitutes, and other multitudes become mothers during their evil career. If the race of the people is of no concern to the State, then has the State no interest in arresting its vitiation. But if this concern and this interest be admitted, then arises the necessity for depriving prostitution not only of its moral, but of its physical venom also. . . .

Success has already attended the introduction of the Act, and I hope my readers will agree with me that the advantages of the Act have been so marked as to induce them to give it an impartial trial in England. From the disinclination to support brothels (in which girls are farmed out) in England, we may hope that our success will be even greater than on the Continent. . . . I have a reasonable belief that if proper legislative measures are taken, clandestine prostitution will be robbed of many of its worst features, and although we may never be able altogether to prevent all its evil effects, we may so far ameliorate it as to render them much less detrimental to society, as well as to the female herself. Let our opponents recollect that if we do not eradicate prostitution, its consequences will remain as a deterrent cause to prevent promiscuous fornication, and this will be in the opinion of some, a great advantage to society. . . .

Assuming that the necessity of State interference will be conceded, that the House of Commons will decide on extending the Contagious Diseases Act to the civil population, let us next consider how the Act may be best worked, by contrasting the past mismanagement with what should be done in future.

It is now many years ago since I called public attention to the error committed by philanthropists and medical men in treating prostitutes as out-patients. I regret to say that what I wrote and published twelve years ago, applies equally to the present day, regarding our civil hospital arrangements. I, however, now go further, and venture to question whether it is desirable for our civil hospitals to treat prostitutes as out-patients at all.

It is matter of very serious regret that the officers of the civil hospital are obliged, from week to week throughout the year . . . to make out-patients of a number of destitute women, whose segregation until cured is imperatively called for by every consideration of public health and morality. I need hardly say that this would not occur were the funds under their control as expansive as their anxiety to diffuse the blessings of the institution; but as it is well known that their large revenues are already fully bespoken and worthily expended, it would be unbecoming in me not to repudiate on their behalf the slightest suspicion of shortcoming. . . .

The propriety and the utility of treating primary symptoms in prostitutes while they remain out-patients seem alike questionable. One, for instance, grievously afflicted, . . . attracted my particular notice by the superiority of her dress. She lived, she said, in her own lodgings in a street near the Strand. It is therefore clear she had no home to look to but the streets unless she paid her rent. In the course of the very same evening I was shocked to see this woman, accompanied by another, soliciting (as the Act of Parliament has it) in the street, and to reflect how frightfully she must contaminate any unfortunate man who might yield to her desperate entreaties. In dress and bearing she was by no means a female of the lowest class. No ordinary observer would have recognized her sanitary condition; but there she was – her rent, her food, her clothes to be earned – obliged to drink intoxicating liquor with every man who might offer it, dangerous alike to gentle and simple, the fast young man, or the tipsy father of a family who might be attracted by her pleasing face, and utterly heedless how much she was protracting, perhaps aggravating, her own sufferings. How comparatively futile our morning labours! how inefficacious the eleemosynary drugs!

Advocates of the 'know-nothing' system, stand aghast! and ask yourselves if the toleration by society of this emissary of death in the occupation in which I saw her is reconcilable with society's duties (if duties it has) to God or man.

Here you see a woman who, patched up by voluntary charity in the morning, knows no other way – nay, whose only possible resource – to get her necessary food, or bed at night, is to sally forth into the streets. The ministers of charity eased her pain this morning; they dressed her sores and gave her drugs. So they will again next Thursday. She may be worse then, or she may have made a little progress in spite of her drinking and her fornication. But in a month she will be no nearer soundness than had she been taken care of by the State within the walls of the hospital for one week; and within that month what a scourge upon society will the surgeons not have kept afoot by their exertions? Here is the power of charity again working to waste. I will not insult you by supposing that you would have had that creature, and the hundreds of whom she is the example, spurned from the gates of every workhouse and hospital, and kicked from every domicile in the name of religion, to perish how and where they might, by lingering, loathsome disease. That were too absurd. But what you do, virtually, is this: You who, if your principles have any worth in them, should protest against the Lock Hospital, proclaim the foul ward a misappropriation, and excommunicate all who relieve or sympathize with the venereal pariah – you neither protest, nor proclaim, nor excommunicate. You testify against none of these things on principle, but only against their extension – against exchanging for a useful flame that inefficient rush-light of private charity which now serves only to make misery visible.

If you consider it wicked encouragement of vice and countenance of immorality to feed, to clothe, to lodge the syphilitic, you will be satisfied that in these . . . cases the hospital administration steered clear of these greater sins. But, though you dare not go so far as to claim the entire dismission of these wretches down the winds of fate, you ought surely, in justice to your principles, to some extent to censure those who wrestled with corruption for their poor bodies, preserved them yet a little longer to defile the earth; perverted charity from what you would allow to be proper objects, and as it were 'threw physic to the dogs'. In truth, we are at a deadlock, all of us – hospital authorities, social Radicals, and social Tories.

The same necessity of selection which is imposed upon the house-surgeon by the restricted number of beds at his disposition, works evil also in another way. As long as it is guided, not by philosophical considerations of public morals and public health, but by that sympathy for suffering humanity which animated the munificent founders of our hospitals, and the proper desire of the medical schools to secure the supervision of the most peculiar forms of disease, we shall take as in-patients only those most malignant and complicated cases, wherein the subject is practically incapable of getting about, and thus, by inference, of earning his or her bread. Thus competition among cases is as it were invited, the premium of a bed is held out for successful severity, and it is no exaggeration to say that the invitation is responded to, and the prize contended for, by the unfortunate out-patients who find themselves from week to week 'not eligible through seniority', 'not yet bad enough' to be taken into the house. The devices, therefore, to which they frequently resort, in order to qualify, are, first to throw away the hospital medicines, and then, reckless of consequences to society, to pursue the best known means of aggravating disease – viz., drunkenness, debauchery, and utter self-neglect.

If the British public could only once conceive the idea that the treatment, cure, and temporary segregation of the syphilitic, was as much a matter of public interest as that of the lunatic, whose seclusion all counties, towns, and parishes provide for with such remarkable alacrity, not so much out of love or respect for him as because he is a dangerous thing to be at large, I think I should not long be alone in wishing for equally public recognition of both complaints. The attitude of society towards those afflicted must, of course, differ; for, whereas upon the former we may properly, I think, exercise compulsion, we can do no more with the other than offer inducements and invitation to be made whole.

Were those inducements ample, in the shape of accommodation and treatment, and were the germs of pestilence sought out with more anxiety than the old neglected cases which are so interesting to the medical classes, we should in a few years have reduced the virulence of hospital syphilis to the level of that now seen in private practice, and of the latter, again, I have no doubt, to a corresponding extent.

* * *

If (in spite of these remarks) prostitutes should still continue to be admitted in the present manner, would it not be well for the civil authorities in future, to exact on admission a promise from them; that they will not of their own free will leave the institution till pronounced cured by the surgeons?

It may be in the recollection of my readers, that some years ago it was given in evidence that prostitutes who were lying in hospitals suffering from venereal diseases, at Portsmouth (on being sent for by the brothel-keepers) on the occasion of a ship being paid off, one and all left their beds to participate in the drinking and rioting that was a necessary consequence, to the no small detriment of her majesty's jolly tars, who of course became affected with the most serious forms of disease. This, I may add, took place before the Contagious Diseases Act came into force, and compulsory residence in hospital (as now enforced) was carried out.

What happened, however, at Portsmouth will necessarily happen in any other place whenever the temptation occurs, or a like inducement is held forth to the patients.

* * *

Having established hospitals, the next question is as to the alterations which may with advantage be made in some of their arrangements, and among other important reforms I would suggest that

Venereal Wards should not be public. That it is desirable for a few pupils to witness all the forms of venereal disease met with among prostitutes, admits of no doubt; I need not say how especially necessary it is that those who propose becoming attached to hospitals and prisons, as well as those who aspire to military, naval, or poor-law appointments, should be well acquainted with these affections. I, however, think it undesirable that the wards wherein a number of diseased unfortunates are confined should be open, as now, to all pupils alike. In lunatic hospitals, selected pupils are alone allowed to enter the wards, and precautions are taken against the abuse of this privilege, the wards being only open to these students, during the visit of the medical man, who gives lectures on the most interesting forms of disease.

In Paris the wards of the female venereal hospitals are so sealed to impertinent curiosity, that a pupil desirous of studying these complaints must become attached to the house in the capacity of *externe*, by special permission of the General Hospital Board, and on the recommendation of the surgeon. He gives his services, whatever they may be worth, in consideration of a daily mess and a stipend of eight francs a month, and has, no doubt, great opportunities of studying disease. An extremely limited number of men, and those selected, therefore, are seen at any time about the wards of the Lourcine Hospital; and as they invariably exhibit the greatest delicacy and politeness towards the unfortunate inmates, such satisfactory relations are maintained between the patients and the doctor as make the word hospital, one of far less horror to French prostitutes than to those of the class in this country.

If no other change is practicable in the system of managing our civil hospitals, I might at least suggest that the crowds of pupils who frequent them should be only allowed to witness the treatment of a selected number of these cases. The inspection of a number of women whose cases present no marked features of interest, can be fraught with no advantage to science, and is painful and demoralizing to the unhappy patients.

Classification of Female Patients. We might, I think, take with advantage another hint from our Continental neighbours, by dividing the women who apply for the cure of venereal complaints into the following classes:

1. The married, who, guiltless themselves, have been injured by their husbands. These are annually becoming more numerous in the London hospitals, and no less than six of them were discharged from the Devonport Lock Hospital in the five months ending May 1869. To compel them, if they enter, to mingle with the hardened offenders, is a scandal to decency and morality, a cruelty to them if they submit to it, if they cannot, a withholding of the means of health.

2. Girls who have been recently seduced and defiled – for their reformation is not hopeless, but often accomplished where proper classification takes place, as in the Lourcine, but is next to impossible if they are placed among the thoroughly vicious, who are too apt to pass their time in hospitals, even when strictly watched, in obliterating all trace of modesty from their less hardened fellow-sufferers.

187

PROSTITUTION

3. Pregnant prostitutes, or those with children – for the child is a certain link between the mother and morality, during the existence of which her case is never hopeless; and charity, placing youth by the side of corruption, has much to answer for.

4. The childless, barren, and confirmed prostitutes.

Among other plans for the amelioration of prostitution which I think it desirable to consider is that of

MIDNIGHT MEETINGS

Various philanthropic individuals have tried the plan of holding midnight meetings in rooms contiguous to the haunts of vice. Sorry should I be to appear even to slight the efforts of any fellow-labourer, but truth compels me to say that of all the useless expedients adopted for remedying by private measures public wrong, this seems about the worst. Such public exhibitions and appeals to excited feelings are scarcely calculated to produce durable impressions.

That which midnight meetings seldom achieve, the proposed medical inspections and hospital detentions ensure, namely access, and in addition they afford the prostitute temporary repose from excitement and time for reflection. These are the very advantages that are attempted to be supplied by Lock asylums and penitentiaries. Notwithstanding the most constant and self-denying exertions of the managers of these institutions, comparatively few fallen women come under their cognizance, and of these very few are permanently reformed.

The following is an admirable description of a midnight meeting, from the *Star* of February 23, 1868:

THE MIDNIGHT MISSION. The enterprises of philanthropy are as varied as its spirit is comprehensive – the means it adopts as flexible as its aim is fixed. The promoters of that new movement which takes the shape of a midnight mission to fallen women do not seek publicity for themselves; but, as they must hope for support from public sympathy and approval, neither do they shroud their doings from the observation of such as may fairly claim to be eyewitnesses. It was at our own instance and request we were on Tuesday night permitted to be spectators of that second gathering at a West-end restaurant of which a brief account appeared next morning. We propose to describe exactly what we saw; and leave to our readers the formation of an impartial, though it cannot be an unsympathizing, judgment.

The invitations distributed in the public resorts of that unhappy class for which we have no name, one does not shrink from writing, fixed twelve o'clock as the hour of meeting. Half an hour past that time, passing up the Haymarket, one could observe a diminution of the usual throng. Midnight is the hour of high-tide on that reef of ship-wrecked souls. When the casinos and music-rooms close, their occu-pants – except the few whose broughams roll them westward to abodes of more secluded vice – flood the adjacent pavements, and gradually subside into the taverns, cafés, and supper-rooms, where paramours may be found or awaited. Tonight there was another and a purer meeting-place open to as many as would enter. Round the door a group of men and youths had formed – curiosity, let us hope, their worst motive and sentiment; for the most unmanned by sensuality would scarcely venture to mock at, or hope to frustrate, the purpose of that gathering. Passing the strictly-guarded entrance, we find ourselves within a room, lofty, spacious, and well furnished. On the tables are tea and coffee, with light comestibles, and nearly every chair has its female occupant. A hundred and fifty of the invited are already present. A dozen or twenty gentlemen, all of mature age, and chiefly in clerical habiliments, are moving about from table to table, and aiding the professional waiters in their duty.

A glance across the room would scarcely reveal the character of the assembly. Are these the 'gay' and the 'unfortunate' – the dashing courtesans or the starveling prostitutes of the West-end? They differ very little in appearance and demeanour from as many women of 'the middle and lower middle class', to adopt Mr Gladstone's discriminat-ing phrase – taken promiscuously. With few exceptions, there are no extravagant dresses – still less are there any symptoms of levity or indecorum. Gravely and quietly, with self-respect and silent courtesy, the refreshments provided are consumed or declined, and newcomers provided with places till not a vacant seat remains. There is one young woman sitting apart, a patriarchal-looking gentleman bending over her, endeavouring, apparently, to console her grief – which, did we not know her vocation and his, we might attribute to the loss of that friend or relative for whom she wears mourning. Here and there is one whose veiled or averted face indicates something of shame or disquietude; but the great majority wear an aspect of cheerful gravity that sets the observer thinking painfully how hearts thus masked may be approached. At least fifty more have entered since we first took note, and the room is crowded to the door; some of the later comers have an air of social outlawry not so marked before, and bold-faced women in silk stand by the side of fellow-sinners in humbler raiment. The disparity of age strikes one more than before. Here are mere girls – girls of sixteen or seventeen – girls who, if seen in pure and happy homes, would have recalled the poet's image of innocent white feet touching the stream that divides childhood from womanhood – girls on whose fair faces paint and drink have not yet replaced the natural bloom with streaks and patches. Here are women of the age at which wise men seek loving helpmates, and children are born early enough to be the pillars of household happiness. And here, too, are women in their ripened prime – women who should be rejoicing, under any burden of domestic care, in the strong arm of a husband's trust and the golden girdle of sons and daughters – but women whose still healthful frames and comely features speak but of a physical vigour invulnerable to twenty years of dissolute pleasure and precarious livelihood. It is a heart-saddening thought that the youngest of these two hundred women is already old in vice – has crossed the line that can never be repassed – has loosed that zone of purity which no power even in Heaven can reclasp. But that to the oldest and most obdurate there is tonight to be offered such help as God or man can give – help that may make the past less terrible by making the future hopeful – it would seem a cruel trifling with human sympathies to collect these victims of irremediable error before eyes that look daily on virtuous wives, and on children that make visible the doctrine, 'heaven lies round about us in our infancy'.

It is about one o'clock when the gentlemen whose activity we have described, gather in a central space on the floor, and one of them requests attention. It is the Hon. and Rev. Baptist Noel who does this – the man who threw up good chances of a bishopric to become a Dissenting pastor.[48] 'My young friends,' he begins; and he has no reason to complain of want of attention, though there are no signs of special interest. He tells his strange audience of that midnight meeting of the two Apostles and their gaoler – the earthquake, and the cry for salvation. He rapidly and plainly applies the story not so much to the conscience as to the consciousness of his hearers. If we had expected that the speaker would so err as to sermonize, we should be happily disappointed. He does not avoid these most deep-seated truths of human duty and destiny which are the basis of religious emotion, but he does not dwell on them. He speaks like a man in the flesh, though not like a man of the world. If he were the latter, he would scarcely warn these comfortable-looking, healthy women that ten years of their present life will send them all to the grave. But there is a hearty human and almost fatherly tenderness in the emphasis he lays on the unreality of their joys, the bitterness of their reflections, the vileness of their seducers, the unworthiness of their habitual associates. He contrasts all this with the possibilities, not only of what they have lost, but of what they may regain. He offers the means of instant rescue – a home, which he takes care to assure them is not a prison; a home in which they shall be subjected to no indignity or privation, but from which they may emerge respected, perhaps beloved. He tells them of others who have thus been saved from all the misery of a sinful life. He refers to a letter from one who, forty years ago, escaped back into good repute, and has grown up in honourable married life. But all this, while he has spoken to an audience more attentive than interested, and certainly not affected. As by an afterthought, he mentions that, since their last meeting, some mother has sent him a photograph of her daughter, be-seeching him to seek that lost one in this company. In an instant the sealed-up fountains are opened, and strong emotion replaces real or feigned indifference. They who heard unmoved of Divine love and human help are touched and shaken by the voice of a weeping mother. Some sob audibly in their tempest of awakened memory. Tears run down the cheeks of many. It seems as though every fallen daughter were asking. 'Is it my mother? Is it my picture?'

Mr Noel is either not an orator, and does not know the power he has gained, or he has reasons for not retouching the chord which so loudly vibrates. Perhaps he wisely desires to avoid any approach to the physical phenomena of revivalism. Yet he might surely use the only key that opens these hearts he so much desires to enter. He resumes his former tone of general exhortation – an impressive and persuasive tone, we should say, did we not see how soon these fair faces have resumed their calm insensibility. He gives way to the Rev. Mr Bickersteth – a clergyman who cannot rid himself of pulpit phrases, but who speaks with an earnest humanity that should make any phraseology a power to melt and move.[49] When he ceases, prayer is offered by Mr Brock, another Baptist minister, and one whose very face is eloquent of kind-hearted goodness.[50] His supplication is surely not unaccompanied. Church congregations are not more decorous than this – let us hope, not more devout. Nearly every face is covered, and some knees are bent. It is such a prayer as every human being can join in – the fervent breathing, in homely words, of a heart that asks aid from Heaven to abate the sin and misery on earth; the sin and misery here, close at hand. . . .

Mr Brock then announces, with loud and cheerful voice, that fifty – a hundred, any number – who will at once quit their present way of life, may this very night be taken to a reformatory home; and if any would return to parents at a distance, the means shall be provided. How many will go? How many will *not* go? we should rather say. Will not all embrace with glad gratitude this proffered rescue? Can any one of these girls and women, who have been for two hours at least restored to the company of good and honourable men and women (for two or three of the latter have aided) – can anyone deliberately go back to the trade and the society that debases and destroys? Alas, yes! Here is one, young and very fair, who replies with a firm though courteous voice, she has decided; and she will not go with the real friends who are now earnestly talking, in groups or singly, with their departing guests. With one exception, and that instantly hushed by her companions, there has been no rude refusal – but there are many who hesitate, and hesitate till they are again lost. Everyone going out seems like a captive carried off by the devil from good angels. But some twenty or more do remain, and over these, whatever chances and changes may await them on the hard road of repentance – over these may we not already rejoice, as does the good shepherd over sheep recovered from the wilderness to the fold?

THE LOCK ASYLUM

My desire to visit the Lock Asylum was gratified by Mr James Lane, surgeon to that institution, who kindly accompanied me through the wards. . . . The buildings are large and lofty, situated a little out of town on the Harrow Road, having been rebuilt within comparatively a few years. It appears that an asylum is offered to all the girls who enter the Lock Hospital, or who are sent there by Government to be cured of venereal diseases under the Contagious Diseases Act. It cannot, however, be said that these poor patients show any great disposition to enter the asylum. In the year 1867, out of 877 patients 76 only entered the asylum, or in other words 8·09 per cent. . . .

The women on admission to the asylum are placed apart in a probationary ward; as we entered this room we noticed fourteen sitting round a table, with the matron at the head, occupying themselves with needlework. In reply to my inquiries I was informed that the latest comer had only been a week in the institution, another had nearly worked out her full probationary period of three months, the rule of the institution being that those who conduct themselves well for that time may become permanent inmates of the institution, in which they can remain for a term varying from twelve to eighteen months, and at the end of it a situation is found for them. In answer to my further inquiries I was told that of twenty who had entered this probationary ward during the preceding six weeks, six had desired to be discharged. I can readily believe that the monotonous life of that ward must have been very irksome to the sort of female habits I have described in the second chapter of this work. The inmates are allowed to walk every day in a sort of courtyard behind the asylum, and are instructed in reading in classes, but I was told that writing is forbidden as leading to correspondence with the outdoor world. Once a month they are permitted to write to their friends, but their letters must be shown to the matron before being put into the post. In another large room we saw twenty-one women working at their needle. These had passed through their probationary period, and I was told might converse quietly as they sat at their work, provided they did not talk loud, another matron, who was seated at the table, constantly supervising them. My informants told me that the matrons objected to sewing machines, having so many human machines to do their work, though, judging from their manner of working, needlework seemed to form but a small share of attention in the institution. I was next taken to the laundry, which seems the staple business of the asylum. In a large, lofty, well-ventilated ground floor, we saw about twenty girls ironing.

Monday and Tuesday in the week, the clothes collected from private families in London are here washed, and at the time of my visit on Thursday the linen was being got up. The matron told me that she thought it took ten months to educate a girl to this business. I asked if there was not a great demand in all parts of the country for laundry-women, having elsewhere heard that it is very difficult for

G

county families to obtain such servants even at high wages; but it appeared that this was not the destination of these girls, who were placed out in small families, where their future career could be watched. It occurred to me, however, that the education of the laundry opened a good career for this class of women.

The Lock Asylum was, at the time of my visit, about half self-supporting. Government provided for ten beds by contributing £20 per bed towards the maintenance of the inmates. The dormitories are excellently constructed. They are lofty rooms, divided by partitions open at the top, and strict rules are laid down for preserving the privacy of each compartment. Whilst passing through the asylum, I asked myself what class of girls do these fifty-two that I see in the wards represent. In the first place, they are the picked and selected of a very large class. These fifty-two women voluntarily come into the asylum. They were the well-behaved, quiet, domesticated, but delicate-looking prostitutes. Making every allowance for the plainness of their dress, as a man of the world I should say that they were not likely to gain a livelihood by prostitution, and I asked myself, as I have done on more than one previous occasion, would not these girls, even if no asylum had been offered to them, have soon left the paths of prostitution and taken to some other calling, merely from their unfitness to undergo its hardships.

If, however, I am at issue sometimes with the authorities of these institutions as to the sort of girl who enters an asylum, I likewise occasionally differ from them as to the way they carry out their philanthropic mission. I was lately visiting a hospital, and the authorities told me that if the girl wished to return to her friends after being cured, not only was the wish seconded, but a policeman was sent with her to see that she really was remitted to the care of her parents.

The plan may be a very good one, to prevent the prostitute being waylaid as she left the hospital by some of her old associates, but it did not seem to occur to the would-be benefactors of the girl that the arrival of a parishioner in charge of a policeman creates a great sensation in a little country community. They did not seem to have contemplated the possibility of the fact that the villagers become curious to learn what Mary Smith has been doing at ——; I ventured to suggest to the authorities that the village gossips would probably over their tea hint at her gay doings, and that the young men would not long be idle in ferreting out her antecedents; and the quiet village, notwithstanding all the care of the rector or aid of his good wife, would be made very disagreeable for the fair penitent who had once quitted her home on an evil errand, and it too often happens she will quit it again, no more to return to her native place.

These bucolic ways are very curious. Let a girl be seduced by one in her own rank, let her have a child, or even two, and her 'misfortune'* may be overlooked, but the parish cannot forgive her having been a gay woman or a soldier's trull. Public opinion, even in a remote country village, has some very curious phases, and I venture to doubt whether its inhabitants cordially take to returned convicts or repentant prostitutes. Sudden reformation is again one of those popular delusions that I must expose. The consequences of vice are not thus to be got rid of. They may be put out of sight; that is all that we can say of them.

On the other hand, in a quiet country community, let a woman be married, and brought home as the wife of a good workman or labourer, her antecedents may be suspected, doubted, or even well known, but as she is the legal wife of one who is responsible for her acts, she is tolerated, and gradually amalgamates with the others, but even then when her female neighbour's wrath is up, she may be reminded of unpleasant truths, and it may be well that her children should be at school, and not hear more of their mother's antecedents than she is herself ready to tell them. . . .

After my visit to the Lock Asylum, I ventured to suggest . . . a doubt whether this and kindred institutions were adapting themselves to the wants of the day. . . . I have often asked myself the question whether it is really necessary to confine a girl from twelve to eighteen months within the walls of an asylum. How many will remain for so long a time in the institution? When they leave the seclusion which they have become accustomed to, are they better adapted than when they entered, for coping with the temptations outside? Are they not liable again to be tempted, and again to fall

---

* Scene a hayfield. The clergyman addresses Mrs Smith, who is raking behind the cart, 'Well, Mrs Smith, how is Fanny?' 'La, sir! why the baby is dead! so now I says she is quite as good as she was afore.' '*Quite!*' said the Rev. gentleman. This was poor Fanny's second *misfortune* as it is called, and so long as the child died, they considered it in this straw-plaiting village as no *misfortune*.

into evil ways? It should be remembered that selected as I have shown them to be, and admirably trained whilst within the walls of the institution, after leaving the asylum they have still to gain a position before they can marry, and amalgamate with the social ranks. I venture to entertain the opinion that many of the philanthropic persons who established these institutions years ago, did so without having previously studied the natural history, the habits, the wants, the tendencies, and the careers of these women. Now that we are better acquainted with all these circumstances, I must be permitted to express a doubt whether their complete segregation is likely to prove permanently beneficial. The upper class of prostitutes are never met with in asylums, nor are the lower. If there are 50,000 prostitutes in London, we need means to rescue not 100 or 1,000, but 12,000 annually, supposing that a prostitute only follows the calling for four years. My object is to assist the many in rescuing themselves and getting away in a few years from a calling that they must detest. My philanthropic friends, however, still maintain that eighteen months' seclusion is required to eradicate the seeds of vice, and they cannot be induced to see that the money can be laid out better, or that any system should be preferred to the one adopted at the Lock Asylum.

★ ★ ★

One mistaken notion, the fallacy of which I have already exposed, lies at the root of the penitentiary system. The old idea, once a harlot always a harlot, possesses the public mind. Proceeding from this premiss, people argue that every woman taken from the streets through the agency of penitentiaries, is a woman snatched from an otherwise interminable life of sin, whereas I have shown that the prostitute class is constantly changing and 'shifting, that in the natural course of events, and by the mere efflux of time the women composing it become reabsorbed into the great mass of our population – and, in fact, those whom the penitentiaries receive are those who are weary of, or unfit for their work, and in search of some other mode of life. The reasonable course to adopt is to assist the natural course of things; to bear in mind that sooner or later the life of prostitution will be quitted, and that the duty of society is to accelerate so far as possible the change, and in the meantime to bring such influences to bear on abandoned women as shall enable them to pass through their guilty years with as little loss of self-respect and health as possible; how to render the prostitute less depraved in mind and body, to cause her return as soon as possible to a decent mode of living, to teach her by degrees, and as occasion offers, self-restraint and self-denial, to build her up, in short – since join society again she will in any event – into a being fit to rejoin it, is the problem to be solved. Will not this be more easily and satisfactorily accomplished by subjecting all alike to supervision and bringing them into daily contact with healthy thought and virtuous life, than by consigning to wearisome and listless seclusion a few poor creatures snatched at haphazard from the streets?

9

PREVENTION OF PROSTITUTION

... Of the various causes to which I have attributed the presence
among us of prostitution, three especially seem worthy of notice in
this chapter: *seduction*, *evil training*, and *poverty*. It is difficult to
obtain statistics sufficiently accurate or reliable to enable us to assign
with any degree of certainty the proportions in which the causes to
which I have adverted operate in the production of prostitutes. It is
scarcely necessary for my purpose to attempt to do so. It seems
sufficient to point out that these three causes exist, and to say that so
far as prostitution can be traced to causes with which human laws
can directly deal, it is traceable to them. We have then to consider
how far the results of seduction may be made to fall short of a
recourse to prostitution, by what means the early vicious training,
with its attendant horrors, may be put an end to, and how far it is
possible to diminish or relieve poverty and its consequences.

It is customary to argue, that the punishment of seduction cannot
be apportioned in any but the present manner, namely, wholly to
the female, unless where illegitimate offspring result from it, in
which case the State imposes a fine of two shillings and sixpence per
week upon the father. The grounds on which the legislature have
decreed this state of the law are, that the woman, if not always the
most active, is a consenting party. The result is practically that the
consequences to the male being known and finite, thousands of men
annually suffer themselves to be seduced – as the law has it – by
designing women, who sacrifice not only their own future peace of
mind and temporal prospects, but court the scorn of the world and
bodily suffering to gratify inordinate passion. The unfortunate male
is the victim, and by curious perversion the manufacture of prostitutes by female labour is rampant.

This is another painful fiction, which, had I the power, I would
attempt to dissipate. If I could not do so much, I would at least
endeavour to devise a means of strengthening the male resolution.
The next time the bastardy laws come up for consideration, I should

propose inquiry how, while in other respects the mental inferiority of woman continues to be insisted on in all other particulars, she should be held paramount in that of seductive powers. That this is false is proved by the fact that the woman allows the sacrifices and sufferings she incurs to equipoise with those of her seducer. She is acquainted too well beforehand with both, to allow the hypothesis of her total ignorance. In the majority of cases he has plentiful knowledge of precedents; yet she falls. She must, therefore, either be temporarily insane, or permanently weaker minded. Her very liability to siege almost presupposes personal attraction, and personal attractions as naturally ensure vanity. . . . Because, from the day when a man in real earnest first set his wit against her, she was no more able to fly from his fascinating power than the quarry from the falcon, or the rabbit from the snake, but rather met her fate half-way, this strong-minded creature is by law considered the real seducer, and a number of the most estimable people in the world are ever ready to endorse without question this cruel article of the law's belief.

And here, again, must physiology be invoked to help the lawgivers and society to a more just conclusion. It will some day be taken into account I hope, that as (I believe) Coleridge said, the desire is on the side of man, love of approbation on the side of the woman; and law will be amended after deeply comparing the physiology of sinning men, not with that of virtuous, but of fallen women.

* * *

It cannot be denied by anyone acquainted with rural life, that seduction of girls is a sport and a habit with vast numbers of men, married . . . and single, placed above the ranks of labour. The 'keeping company' of the labouring classes, accompanied by illicit intercourse, as often as not leads to marriage; but not so that of the farmer's son, farmer, first, second, or third-class, squire, or squireen. Many such rustics of the middle class, and men of parallel grades in country towns, employ a portion of their spare time in the coarse, deliberate villainy of making prostitutes. Of these, the handsomer are drafted off into the larger communities, where their attractions enable them to settle; the others are tied to the spot of their birth and fall. Men who themselves employ female labour, or direct it for others, have always ample opportunities of choice, compulsion,

secrecy, and subsequent intimidation, should exposure be probable
and disagreeable. They can, for a time, show favour to their victim
by preferring her before her fellows; they can at any convenient
moment discharge her. The lower sort of them can often procure
access to the Union for both her and her offspring; and the upper can
scheme marriages of the nature alluded to at page 74. With these,
and with the gentlemen whose *délassement* [pastime] is the contamination of town servants and *ouvrières* [working women], the first
grand engine is, of course, vanity – the little more money that will
get the poor girl a little more dress, admiration, and envy than her
equals enjoy. Then, when the torch is set to the fire, woman's love
of approbation helps her to her own destruction. Then cheap
promises – promises of marriage – made to be broken – which,
however, the strong-minded one of the Parliament's imagining is
always ready to believe – and promises often taken down on the rolls
of Heaven, whose breach must be a sin against the God of Mercy
himself, of care for the woman and her offspring. But the latter are
as easily snapped as the former, and the woman whom her neighbours call a scheming hussy for thinking of a marriage above her
station, is called a silly fool for her pains if she fall, without inducements of ambition, before the assault of passion only. She may be
with child, or she may not, but she has at law a remedy for her
wrong. Yes, and what is it? Will the strong-minded one apply herself to it? – and how often?

She loved too much, and she still loves overmuch, in nine cases
out of ten, to dream of worldly wisdom, or, as she calls it, persecuting
her child's father. The worldly wisdom that overcame, as the sham
has it, the hardihood and modesty of the male, and turned his head,
cannot get its poor owner into a court of justice, even when her
parents are so minded, and funds are forthcoming for a breach of
promise action. Her remedy is a farce so far; or rather it is a farce
to say that it has any prophylactic or *in terrorem* [warning]
value. But she has one more remedy – or her friends have; for her
father, whom the law supposes to be charged with the maintenance
of his children when derelict by the world, and therefore to have in
return some presumed employer's right over them, may proceed at
common law for loss of her services. But this he can only do if he
has means, inclination to face the extreme of publicity and abuse,
courage to meet a heavy preponderance of law and public feeling

against him, and can adduce an amount of corroborative evidence which should suffice to carry a much more heavy conviction. This machinery, which stands upon a fiction, is cumbrous, and its results are rare and generally ridiculous. It amounts, in fact, to no remedy for wrong; and the crime which it is supposed to check flourishes under its pleasant shade. There is, however, one tolerably certain method of enforcing law against a man who, having seduced, has deserted a woman and her child. When we have recited that, we may close the list of remedies. She may apply to a bench of magistrates for a summons. The summons is granted; and the man found, or not found, the usual result is 'an order in bastardy', in pursuance of which the maximum sum of half a crown is due and payable by the father each and every week for the support and maintenance of the said infant, but for that of his strong-minded seducer – nothing!

Sighing – or, it may be, smiling compassionately at the crestfallen appearance of the strong one who has found hardihood to come before them – the bench of justices regret their inability to do more for her. They would make an example if they could, they say in some instances; in others, they make an order for only 1s. 6d. or 2s. a week. The magistrate, who is a family man, and has perchance himself grown a crop of wild oats, gives a sad thought or two to the case as he jogs home; and has even been known to advocate in public some more extended protection of women. But the plague is for all that – as it may be when I, too, am passed away – yet unstayed. The days of chivalry are gone indeed, and the honour of all women but those of his own house is so much a by-word with the Englishman – their bodies so often his sport – that the reform of the bastardy law, and the thence resulting check to prostitution, may chance to be deferred until a sense of common danger shall have made us all fellow-agitators.

If I could not get imprisonment of the seducer substituted for the paltry fine of half a crown a week, I would at least give to the commonwealth, now liable to pecuniary damage by bastardy, some interest in his detection and punishment. The Union house is now often enough the home of the deserted mother and the infant bastard: and the guardians of the poor ought, I think, to have the right, in the interest of the community, to act as bastardy police, and to be recouped their charges. I would not allow the maintenance of an illegitimate child to be at the expense of any but the father. I would make it the incubus on him, not on its mother; and I would not leave his detection, exposure, and money loss in the option of the latter. A young man who now has a second or third illegitimate child, by different women, has not lived without adding some low cunning to his nature. It often happens that a fellow of this sort will, for a time, by specious promises or presents to a girl he fully intends ultimately to desert, defer making any payments for or on account of her child. If he can for twelve months, and without entering into any shadow of an agreement (and we may all guess how far the craft of an injured woman will help her to one that would hold water), stave off any application on her part to the authorities, her claim at law is barred; and she herself, defied at leisure, becomes, in due course, chargeable to her parish or union. But not thus should a virtuous State connive at the obligations of paternity being shuffled on to its public shoulders, when, by a very trifling modification of the existing machinery they might be adjusted on the proper back – permanently or temporarily, as might be considered publicly expedient.

I would enact, I say, by the help of society, that, in the first place, the seduction of a female, properly proved, should involve the male in a heavy pecuniary fine, according to his position – not at all by way of punishment, but to strengthen, by the very firm abutment of the breeches-pocket, both him and his good resolutions against the temptations and force of designing woman. I would not offer the latter, as I foresee will be instantaneously objected, this bounty upon sinfulness – this incentive to be a seducer; but, on the contrary, the money should be due to the community, and recoverable in the county court or superior court at the suit of the Government Board; and should be invested by the treasurer of such court, or by the county, or by some public trustee in bastardy, for the benefit of mother and child. The child's portion of this fund should be retained by such public officer until the risk of its becoming chargeable to the community quasi bastard should be removed by the mother's marriage, or otherwise; and the mother's share should be for her benefit as an emigration fund or marriage portion. Persons acquainted with the country will bear me out, that many a woman not married by her seducer for economy's sake (which would satisfy justice), would, with a dower, even thus accruing, soon re-enter the pale of society through the gate of matrimony. I think that very useful knowledge of such a law as this would be rapidly diffused, and be found materially to harden men's hearts against female seductions.

Morality based on fear has, I grant, a most rotten foundation. But the reader must remember that the ear and heart of man, once barred by salutary caution against the charmings of all save exceptional and ungovernable lust, would be much more accessible to the moralizing influence – the legitimate attachment – which I have proposed that society should simultaneously hold out at a cheaper rate. To the practical, systematic seducer – no uncommon character – upon whom moral argument is, and always will be, thrown away, this pursuit would, under such a régime, become a very first-class and most expensive luxury, demanding more money, craft, and time than many of us have to dispose of.

* * *

A glance at the returns made by the Registrar-General, of the causes of death among infant bastards, is sufficient to prove that a large proportion perish from neglect or improper treatment. Such headings as the following cannot fail to attract notice, and seem to point their own moral: 'Accidental suffocation', 'suffocated in bed', 'lying on its face', 'accelerated by cold', 'want of maternal nourishment', 'want of breast milk', 'low vitality', 'marasmus',[51] 'atrophy', 'emaciation', 'gradual wasting from birth', 'exhaustion from diarrhoea'.

The following instance of a baby contract shows the sort of terms on which the transfer of infants can be effected, and the sort of care that the adopting party can be reasonably expected to bestow.

Mr Bedford, the coroner for Westminster, held an inquiry at the Charing Cross Hospital, on the body of Fanny Williams, aged eight months. Mrs Brown, the wife of a gilder, living at 1, Plough-yard, Crown-street, Soho, said that about four months ago she had taken charge of and adopted the child from its mother, a single woman, named Caroline Williams. On Thursday night last she was sitting in her room with the child on her lap, when it was suddenly seized with convulsions. She at once took it to Dr Cooper, of Moor-street, who advised her to take it to the hospital. She did so, but on its arrival it was pronounced by the house surgeon to be dead. Caroline Williams, aged seventeen, the mother of the child, said she was a single woman.

She was confined with the deceased child in June last. She had saved a few pounds in service, and being unable to attend properly to her child, she answered an advertisement she saw in a paper, from a Mrs Brown, who desired to adopt a child. She saw Mrs Brown on the subject, and after some conversation together, Mrs Brown agreed to adopt her child for £5, and the following agreement was drawn up: 'Received of Caroline Williams £5, for which sum I agree to take and adopt her child, Fanny Williams, and to bring it up in a respectable manner; failing to do which I agree to forfeit and pay to the said Caroline Williams the sum of £20. The said child to be no further trouble or expense to its mother or friends – Ann Brown.' She had never seen her child since. The medical evidence showed that the child was brought in dead on Thursday last. It had died from convulsions, brought on by teething. There was no reason to suppose the child had not been properly nourished, or unfairly treated. The coroner having remarked upon the extraordinary document which had been put in by the mother, and condemned the system of advertising for children, a verdict of death from natural causes was returned.

I have said enough to show the horrors of this atrocious system. It would be to little purpose to accumulate anecdotes and instances. If the reader will apply to the plain statement of facts and results that I have given his own common sense and experience of human nature, he can picture for himself the evils that must of necessity result, especially when we remember that the moral and religious training bestowed upon such of these poor children as may survive in spite of neglect, cruelty, and privation, is likely to be on a par with the attention and care bestowed upon their physical and sanitary requirements. We may now turn to the other results of seduction and desertion . . .: concealment of birth and infanticide. . . .

A learned writer has remarked upon the small amount of crime convicted when compared with the amount of crime committed.* His remark is made with reference to forgers, thieves, and others who fall strictly under the designation criminal classes. It is, however, also true, though perhaps in a less degree, of the forms of evil now under consideration, that the amount of crime detected forms but a small proportion of the crime committed. We must bear this in

* Hill, *Suggestions for the Repression of Crime* (1857), 7.

mind when referring for information on the state of the public morals to the judicial statistics. Were it otherwise, we might read with some complacency that the cases of infanticide were in the year 1865, when the numbers of births of legitimate children amounted to 701,484 and of illegitimate to 46,585, only 83, and that the endeavours to conceal births were according to the same returns no more than 209 in 1867, 211 in 1866, and 222 in 1865. When, however, we pass on to the returns of the Registrar-General, we shall find that the appearance of things is far less satisfactory. In the year 1865 no less than 199,810 deaths of infants under one year old are reported, or more than half of the total of infants perishing under the age of five years. Of these deaths, 183 are attributed to homicide, against 198 so perishing under five years; in other words, of 198 babies murdered before attaining five years of age, all but fifteen were less than a year old. Of these latter the total number of violent deaths occurring in 1865 is returned at 1,698, of which 1,447 are attributed to accident or negligence, and 165 are unclassed. In addition to these 1,698 deaths confessedly violent, we find 699 under the heading, sudden causes unknown, and 2,710 under the equally suspicious heading of causes not specified. These returns will do much to modify any complacency that we may have contracted while perusing the judicial statistics, especially when we remember that the cases of concealment of birth are usually cases of infanticide also, but included in the milder category by the leniency of judges and juries.

It may be said that black as this list of deaths confessedly is, there is nothing to show that it is confined to the illegitimate, and that brutality is well known to be confined to no set of people in particular, and to be found among parents who have availed themselves of the rites of the church previously to living together, as well as among those who have neglected or despised them. A little consideration will, I think, suffice to satisfy the inquirer that a vast majority of the artificially accelerated deaths fall upon infants born outside the married pale. It will be remembered, that the proportion of bastard to legitimate children is about six per cent, that is, that for every child resulting from unlawful embraces, sixteen are produced by the marriage bed. Bearing these figures in mind, we shall receive vast instruction from a perusal of the coroner's returns.

A little . . . examination of the figures at our disposal seems to place almost beyond the possibility of doubt the supposition that a large proportion of the illegitimate children brought into the world meet with a violent, or at least premature end. We find that the number of inquests held on illegitimate children of the age of one year, but under seven, amounted to 2,960, while the number held upon legitimate children of a like age reaches only to 201. There is here a preponderance of illegitimate deaths striking enough to call forth suspicions of foul play. . . . It is at the outset of the baby's life that the mother has to answer for herself whether she can bear the shame that must inevitably occur to her from that infant life. During that evil time, also, it becomes apparent whether or no the father will support the life he called forth, and whether, if he fails to take the burden on himself, the mother can make up by her exertions for his default. Let the first gust of shame pass over, the first difficulty of providing for the babe be faced and overcome, and it is reasonable to suppose that the chances against its life being preserved are little greater than those against the attainment to maturity of the offspring of married life.

The results, then, of seduction and desertion are to force the mother to take to prostitution, and to tempt her to make away with her child either by her own hand or by means of baby farmers, thus giving rise to an amount of crime fearful to contemplate, while if the children survive the neglect and ill-treatment of their early years, can it be hoped that they will do otherwise than swell the ranks of the pauper and criminal classes?

★　★　★

Under the present bastardy laws the mother must be the applicant for redress, and the interference of others, either in her interest or in that of the ratepayers, is not tolerated; while the right allowed her of claiming, previously to the birth of the child, the assistance of the magistrate, is seldom or never acted upon, and virtually a dead letter. The advantage that would accrue from the exercise of this right is self-evident; so great is it, that it should not merely be permitted as a right, but imposed as an obligation. That the person interested in concealing the birth, and desirous of screening the father, even to her own and her infant's hurt, should be the only one by whom action can be taken, is a gross absurdity. If the injury consequent on her silence recoiled on herself alone, it might be unfair to take from her the opportunity for self-sacrifice; but she cannot suffer alone; her helpless babe, and the whole community, suffer from her mistaken lenity. The right to set in motion the machinery of the law against the father should be extended to other persons. There are few women more exposed to temptation to immorality than domestic servants, especially those serving in houses where men servants also are kept; if the pregnancy of any such servant comes to the knowledge of her master, he should have the right allowed to him of making her condition known to the magistrates, and taking the steps necessary for ensuring the detection of her paramour – nay, more, the adoption of this course should be made obligatory upon him, and he might be made answerable for any miscarriage of justice arising from his wilful default by being himself made chargeable to the same extent as the putative father would have been but for his neglect. The same principle might be adopted in the case of shopkeepers and other employers of female labour. Such a course would obviate the evils arising under the present system; a woman found pregnant is usually dismissed from her employment without a character; and yet the adoption of this course is ruin to her, and affords her seducer an additional chance of escaping the consequences of his wrong-doing. Were her dismissal accompanied by the further action here suggested, her first false step would be no longer irretrievable, and the author of her shame would be made a partner in her responsibilities. We are too apt in this utilitarian and self-seeking age to forget that incidental, as well as direct, duties attend the different social relationships.

* * *

Closely akin to the relief of the seduced woman and the prevention of her further fall is the amelioration and reformation of the prostitute. . . . I have little faith in the efficacy of lock asylums and penitentiaries; nor from the agency of enforced seclusion do I anticipate reformation, but from the gradual instilling of sentiments of self-respect and self-restraint. I therefore do not advocate the establishment of penitentiaries on a large scale, but 'by line upon line, and precept upon precept, here a little and there a little', good may be done to these unfortunate outcasts. It is the only plan, gradually to educate them back to a sense of decency. Practical men devoting their time and thoughts to the carrying out of a special object, and learning from the experience and from the mistakes no less than

207

from the successes of the past, wisdom for the future, are more likely to hit upon the means of solving a difficult problem than mere theorists or amateurs. I would, therefore, entrust to this board the carrying out of the Contagious Diseases Act, and vest in it power to make such provision as should from time to time seem expedient to assist in the paths of reformation, such women as on leaving the hospital, or from any other cause, should desire to abandon prostitution. The funds of the board would consist of the property held at present by the Foundling Hospital, and of such further sums raised either by parliamentary grant or parochial rates, as might be necessary. The funds thus vested in it, and the sums recovered from the fathers of bastards, together with the profits arising from the employment of the women received into the institution, would go far towards defraying its expenses, and any additional sums required would contribute to lighten the public burdens in other ways, and therefore form no additional charge upon the ratepaying and taxpaying population.

If we can by this means, or in any other way prevent seduced women from becoming, and their daughters from growing up into prostitutes, we shall, if our position be true – that the supply stimulates and increases, and to a certain extent creates the demand – have taken a great preventive step. There is more, however, that we may do – we may take care that so far as possible no persons shall be permitted to follow any calling that makes them interested in the continuance and increase of prostitution, and the procuring a supply of prostitutes; further, that prostitutes shall ply their trade in a manner as little degrading as possible. For these two reasons the trade of a brothel-keeper must be resolutely put down.

★   ★   ★

Having, in the chapter on 'Causes of Prostitution', referred to the vice bred like filth, from the miserable herding of the lower orders, it becomes me also to number the improvement of their dwellings among preventive measures. The passing of the Common Lodging-house Act of 1851, rendering compulsory the registration of such houses and the compliance of their keepers with certain regulations demanded by decency and cleanliness, was a step in the right direction; and the results thereby obtained are satisfactory as showing how much has been done – painful as showing what is still to do.

It is clear that the whole number have not yet been brought under supervision. This must be a work of time; but enough good has resulted hitherto to encourage us to proceed in what is obviously the way of right.

A step above these common lodging-houses are the so-called private dwellings, where each chamber is let to a separate family. These are subject by law to none but health inspections; but their occupants being generally of a class to whom all decency within their means is as grateful as to the wealthiest, the promiscuous crowding is a source of pain to them that the public would further its own interest by helping to alleviate. None can feel more acutely than the working classes of all grades the great difficulty of procuring wholesome dwellings near the seat of their labour. Many men live miles away from their work, in order to preserve their growing families from the moral and physical contamination of the crowded courts and alleys, in which only they could find lodgings within their means. The State by itself, or by energetically putting the screw of compulsion upon the municipalities, who are slow to avail themselves of permissive enactments, to love their neighbours as themselves, should hold out a helping hand to the working million, who are, for want of dwellings adapted to their use, drifting to and fro among the wretched London 'tenements', or reduced to harbour in the common lodging-house.

This packing of the lower classes is clearly not yet under control, and seems liable to aggravation by every new thoroughfare and airway with which we pierce our denser neighbourhoods. While it prevails, who can impute the defilement of girls, the demoralization of both sexes, as blame to the hapless parent who does the best he can with his little funds, and procures the only accommodation in the market open to him? It is preposterous, as I have before hinted, to attribute the prostitution so engendered to seduction, or to vicious inclinations of the woman. From that indifference to modesty, which is perforce the sequel of promiscuous herding, it is a short step to illicit commerce; and this once established, the reserve or publicity of the female is entirely a matter of chance.

Among the preventives that we ought to consider before attempting the *cure* of prostitution, should be numbered an altered and improved system of female training. Some remarks on this point published in *The Times* many years ago, are still extremely pertinent.

When we examine our system of training for girls of the poorer class, we see one very important defect immediately in it, and that is that they receive no instruction in household work. Girls are taught sewing in our parish schools, and very properly, because, even with a view to domestic service, sewing is an important accomplishment; but they are not taught anything about household work. We do not say that a parish school could teach this, for household work can only be really learnt *in* a house; the schoolroom can provide napkins and towels, but it cannot supply tables, chairs, mantelpieces, and carpets for rubbing and brushing; and, the material to work upon being wanting, the art cannot be taught. But this is only explaining the fact, and not altering it. Household work is not learnt, and what is the consequence? The department of domestic service in this country is hardly at this moment sufficiently supplied, while crowds of girls enter into the department of needlework in one or other of its branches, and of course overstock it enormously. Add to this a sort of foolish pride that poor people have in the apparent rise which is gained in rank by this profession – for, of course, every one of these girls is ultimately to be 'a milliner', which has for them rather a grand sound. The metropolis, sooner or later, receives this vast overplus of the sewing female population, and the immense milliners' and tailors' and shirtmakers' establishments hardly absorb the overflowing supply of female labour and skill, while, of course, they profit to the very utmost by the glut of the labour-market. A vast multitude of half-starving women is the result of the system; whereas, had household work formed a part of their instruction, besides a better supply of the home field of service, what is of much more consequence, the colonies would take a large part of this overplus off our hands. . . .

What is the natural remedy, then, for this defect in the training of girls of the poorer classes in this country? The remedy is, of course, that they should be taught in some way or other household work. At present, in the absence of any such instruction as this, it must be admitted that, however incidentally, the sewing which is taught in all our parish schools is simply aiding the overflowing tide of needle labour, which is every year taking up such multitudes of young women to the metropolis, and exposing them to the dreadful temptations of an underpaid service. And how is household work to be taught? Well, that is, of course, the difficulty. There are, as we have said, great difficulties in the way of our parish schools taking it up. The experiment, however, has been tried, in different places, of special institutions for this object; and, in the absence of any formal and public institutions, the houses of our gentry and clergy might be made to supply such instruction to a considerable extent, and without any inordinate demand on private charity. Extra labour, as every householder knows, is often wanted in every domestic establishment; it is even wanted periodically and at regular intervals in a large proportion of our good houses. It would be of great service to the country if a practice, which is already partially adopted, were more common and general – that of taking parish girls by turns for these special occasions. This might be done, at any rate in the country, to a large extent, and even a few days' employment of this kind in a well-furnished house, occurring at more or less regular intervals, would be often enough to create a taste and a capacity for household work. The profession of household service might thus be indefinitely widened, and a large class be created that would naturally look to such service as its distinct employment, and be ready, in case of disappointment at home, to seek it in the colonies.*

I shudder as I read each jubilant announcement of 'another new channel for female labour'. Each lecture, pamphlet, and handbill, that calls attention to some new field of competition, seems to me but the knell of hundreds whose diversion by capital from their natural functions to its own uses, is a curse to both sexes and an hindrance of the purposes of our Creator. No more impious *coup d'État* of Mammon could be devised than that grinding down against one another of the sexes intended by their Maker for mutual support and comfort.

Free trade in female honour follows hard upon that in female labour; the wages of working men, wherever they compete with female labour, are lowered by the flood of cheap and agile hands, until marriage and a family are an almost impossible luxury or a misery. The earnings of man's unfortunate competitor are in their turn driven down by machinery until inadequate to support her life. The economist, as he turns the screw of torture, points complacently to this further illustration of the law of trade; the moralist pointing out how inexorable is the command to labour, too seldom and too late arrests the torture. He only cries enough when the famished

* *The Times*, May 6, 1857.

worker, wearied of the useless struggle against capital, too honest yet to steal, too proud yet to put up useless prayers for nominal relief at the hands of the community, and having sold even to the last but one of her possessions, takes virtue itself to market. And thus, as Parent-Duchâtelet says, 'prostitution exists, and will ever exist, in all great towns, because, like mendicancy and gambling, it is an industry and an expedient against hunger, one may even say against dishonour. For, to what excess may not an individual be driven, penniless, her very existence compromised? This last alternative, it is true, is degrading, but it nevertheless exists.'*

But if the national education of women is not to be confined to reading, writing, and needlework, what are we to do with them? The ready answer is – TEACH THEM HOUSEWIFERY; and the rejoinder, how and where, was well met by the sensible and practical suggestion in the newspaper article above quoted, 'that household education should be incorporated to a much greater extent than at present, with the discipline of Union houses and schools'.

The parochial clergy and well disposed gentry of the country have ample opportunities, if they would embrace them, of diverting to household pursuits the crowds of young women who annually jostle one another into the ranks of needlework. The hall, the parsonage, and the parish school would be the best of normal schools for cooking, scrubbing, washing, ironing, and the like. Their owners would gladly, I fancy, impart gratuitous instruction in exchange for gratuitous service, and every housekeeper will bear me out in saying that the knowledge of the business once acquired, the market for properly qualified domestic servants is ample and not half supplied, while that for every description of needlework has long been overstocked. The vanity of girls and mothers must, it is true, be overcome, but the greater economy of the proposed domestic education would go some way to carry the day in its favour; and if a true appreciation of the happiness that waits on colonization, and of the essentials to its success, were once to get well abroad among our people, their mother wit would lead them soon enough to grasp the comparative value of the domestic and needlework systems of training.

Prostitution, though it cannot be directly repressed, may yet be

* [Parent-Duchâtelet, *De la prostitution dans la ville de Paris*, 3rd edition (1857), I. 339–40. Acton's translation has been amended.]

acted upon in many ways, and in proportion as the social system is wisely administered will its virulence be abated. We cannot put it down, but we can act indirectly on both the supply and demand. A judicious system of emigration will direct into healthy channels the energy that in overpeopled countries finds an outlet in riot, wickedness, and crime. Still, in advocating emigration as helping to prevent the spread of prostitution, I am far from advising that single women should be sent to the colonies alone and unprotected.

★ ★ ★

I have now accomplished my task, but before taking leave of the reader I would press most earnestly upon his mind and conscience the duty of reflecting seriously on the subject to which in these pages I have called attention. We have in the midst of us a great and fearful evil, whose existence is acknowledged and deplored by all, while to the consideration how best we may deal with it, all seem to give the go-by with one consent. I ask, is this right? If I am told that it is a matter that must be left to itself to work its own cure, that as the world grows older it grows wiser, and that the progress of education makes virtue more loved, vice more detested, I ask, is this really so? Does anyone in his heart of hearts believe it? Does the course of passing events lend credit to the hope? Is society growing more virtuous? is it not quite the reverse, and patent to everyone that there is a change passing over it, and that not in the right direction? Lest I should be considered a prejudiced witness, let me call on my behalf one of the most popular journals of the day. In the *Pall Mall Gazette* for the 16th of April, 1869, appeared the following remarkable commentary on the sights to be witnessed daily in the very centre of fashionable life:

The Ladies' Mile. – Although up to this period of the season the people who ride or drive in the Row have not been distracted by any specially sensational ponies under the direction of anonymous ladies, questionable broughams and horsebreakers have even thus early appeared in Hyde Park in excess of the number with which the assemblage is usually enlivened. But it is not so much of this circumstance, however, that we now write. In itself it is bad enough, but it is difficult to see how such people could be kept out of the Parks. There is a significance, however, in another social aspect of the matter which is

213

more important. Until very recently there was no such thing as a *demi-monde* in London, using the term in its imperfect meaning, as understood here. The wretched women went down rapidly from one stage to another without being encouraged or systematized sufficiently to form a regular set – having establishments and holding receptions such as distinguish a corresponding class in Paris. But within a very brief period – not much more than a year, perhaps – there has been a change among us. Previous to that time, indeed, moralists in the press complained of the frank terms which young men of fashion held with such women in places of public resort. This familiarity is now so much on the increase (as anyone who watches what goes on in the Ladies' Mile can perceive) that it calls for some remonstrance.

Formerly Aspasia and her associates were passed with a nod, or only spoken to by men who were indifferent to notice because they were themselves unknown, or, at any rate, if they recognized such women they were cautious where it was done. At present the yellow chignoned denizens of St John's-wood and Pimlico draw up their carriages or horses close to the rails, and are chatted with as candidly as if they had come from some dovecot in the country watched over by a virtuous mother. The audacity of these *réunions* is unprecedented. A notion seems to prevail that the loose women of our own day are undistinguishable from the women of virtue. The superstition is preposterous. In the Park, at least, there is no difficulty in distinguishing the carriage that anybody may pay for, or in guessing the occupation of the dashing *equestrienne* [horsewoman] who salutes half a dozen men at once with her whip or with a wink, and who sometimes varies the monotony of a safe seat by holding her hands behind her back while gracefully swerving over to listen to the compliments of a walking admirer. Of course the men who talk with these women of the highway are perfectly aware of what they are about, and a London lady tempered in the atmosphere of one or two seasons learns discretion enough not to ask relevant questions when she meets in a ball-room the same gentleman she has observed *tête-à-tête* with Aspasia in the Row: If things go on, however, as they seem likely to, this sort of reserve will be tested with unusual severity in the months of May and June.

The manner in which what again, for want of a more convenient phrase, we must call the *demi-monde* class, has been freshly developed among us is not unknown. There are certain perfumers' shops at the West-end notorious for enterprises not immediately connected with bloom for the lips and glitter for the eyes. It was from one of these establishments that a well-known photograph and its original were, so to speak, floated. Here loungers turn in, and are invited to balls, for which cards are given them. Thence spring intimacies of which we say no more than that the acknowledgment of them should be suspended before virtuous women in the Park. The ladies have a remedy in their hands which they deliberately abandon when they pretend blindness to what is as obvious as the Duke's statue at the Corner. And, of course, if they choose to encourage the open and flagrant disrespect to which they are treated there is no help for them.

I appeal with confidence to everyone acquainted with London life, and ask if this statement is not strictly true? but in that case, what becomes of the notion that the mischief, if left to itself, will work out its own cure? I appeal to those who fear God, and reverence His laws, and who therefore refuse to recognize, lest by so doing they should be supposed to countenance, vice, and I ask them to consider whether this attitude of indifference is not open to a construction far different to that which they themselves would put upon it. May not those who follow evil courses say, 'We know that our lives are obnoxious to censure, that the finger of scorn is pointed at us, but the law will not touch us, and why? because it dare not; and it dares not, because whatever good people may think or say to the contrary, our sin, if sin indeed it be, is committed in obedience to natural laws; surely nature's teaching is at least as good as that of religion.'

And so it comes to pass that men consider the sin as a thing that everybody practises, though nobody talks much about it, until to abstain is looked upon almost as a mark of want of manhood, and the natural consequence is that what everybody does nobody feels ashamed to acknowledge participation in, and if such is the state of public feeling, who can be surprised at the condition of things to which attention is called by the article above quoted. Now, I say the time has arrived when serious men should give to prostitution serious thought. It can no longer be ignored. The evils attendant on it are too great and too much on the increase. Evil agents are active and stirring, and those whose lives are pure, who love their country and their fellow men, must show an equal diligence. The field of inquiry may be repulsive, the problems that meet us difficult of solution, and my fellow labourers must expect for a season at least to have only their labour for their pains, and for their only reward an approving conscience. But we may trust that the time is approaching when the justice of our cause will be acknowledged. It cannot be that the people of this country will for ever ignore the misery to be found in their midst. Nor even to human ears can 'the crying of the poor and the sighing of the needy' for ever appeal in vain.

It is absolutely impossible to exaggerate the suffering entailed by a life of prostitution. Instead of the scorn so freely lavished on the poor lost daughters of shame and misery, I plead for a little pity – nay, far more than pity, I plead for justice. If unequal laws between man and woman compel to a shameful and a hated trade the helpless and shuddering victim of seduction, whose fall, though it has soiled and stained, has not utterly polluted her, I charge those laws with cruelty, and I say further that her blood is on the head of those who know the injustice of such laws yet will not help to alter them. If human beings are left to herd together with indecent indiscriminacy, because in this rich and luxurious city they can obtain no more fitting shelter; if they are allowed to grow up from childhood to youth, and from youth to adult years amid scenes of depravity and sin, I ask on whose shoulders does the blame really rest; whether on the victim's, reared to a life of infamy, or on society's, that leaves them to a fate so awful. If in this wide world, teeming with abundant supplies for human want, to thousands of wretched creatures no choice is open save between starvation and sin, may we not justly say that there is something utterly wrong in the system that permits such things to be? If the traffic in human flesh and female honour is not repressed by the arm of the law, may we not justly accuse the law of falling far short of its duty? And if all this be true, is there not abundant cause of prostitution that is capable of removal? Is it too much to say that by amending the bastardy laws, by improving the dwellings of the poor and keeping the young from haunts of vice, by encouraging and promoting emigration, and resolutely putting down so far as possible the great body of night-house keepers and brothel-keepers throughout the country, the number of prostitutes will be greatly decreased? Prostitution we cannot prevent, but we can mitigate the misery entailed by it, and can do much, if we will, to prevent women becoming prostitutes. The evil cannot be done away, but it may be lessened, and that to a very great extent. We cannot do all we wish:

is that a reason for doing nothing? Let us do what we can. The mischief that must always exist will have more or less intensity according as we regulate it, or leave it to itself. The women will become more or less depraved, according as good and healing influences are brought to bear upon, or withheld from them. The numbers who resort to a shameful trade will lessen or increase according as the causes of prostitution are removed or neglected. The neutral position has been fairly tried, but the nation is certainly not improving. Let us assume a position at once more manly and more humane. The evils to be overcome are too intense for individual effort to cope with, but the good which scattered philanthropists, earnest and self-devoted though they be, cannot achieve, is not beyond attainment if wise, discriminating and concentrated power is enlisted in the cause. While men stood with folded arms aghast at the evil which appeared of too long standing, and too stupendous for human power to cope with, the filth of the Augean stables continued to accumulate, but when resolute will, high intelligence, and manly courage took the task in hand, and let loose upon the filthy stalls the cleansing waters, the mischief was removed. Laugh not, neutral reader, at the old classic tale, *'mutato nomine de te fabula narratur'*.

APPENDIX A

THE HAYMARKET IN THE EIGHTEEN-FIFTIES

This description, from Charles Dickens's weekly, Household Words, *is quoted by Acton in a footnote to the section on 'Pleasure Gardens and Dancing Rooms' (see p. 52). The introductory sentence is Acton's.*

Although the aspect of the Haymarket is somewhat improved of late years, its condition is still disgraceful, and the following description of it by Albert Smith,[52] in *Household Words* of the 12th September, 1857, is still, to a great extent, applicable:

About the top of this thoroughfare is diffused, every night, a very large part of what is blackguard, ruffianly, and deeply dangerous in London. If Piccadilly may be termed an artery of the Metropolis, most assuredly that strip of pavement between the top of the Haymarket and the Regent Circus is one of its ulcers. By day, the greater part of the shops and houses betray the character of the locality. Some there are, indeed, respectable; but they appear to have got there by chance, and must feel uncomfortable; the questionable ones preponderate. Observe the stale, drooping lobsters, the gaping oysters, the mummified cold fowl with its trappings of flabby parsley, and the pale fly-spotted cigars; and then look into the chemist's windows, and see, by the open display, in which direction his chief trade tends. Study the character of the doubtful 'people you see standing in doorways – always waiting for somebody as doubtful as themselves – and wonder what the next 'plant' is to be, which they are now cogitating. It is always an offensive place to pass, even in the daytime; but at night it is absolutely hideous, with its sparring snobs, and flashing satins, and sporting gents, and painted cheeks, and brandy-sparkling eyes, and bad tobacco, and hoarse horse-laughs, and loud indecency. Cross to the other side of the way, go out into the mud, get anywhere rather than attempt to force your passage through this mass of evil; for it will most probably happen – as if this conglomeration of foul elements was not enough to stop the polluted stream trying to flow on – that a brass band has formed a regular dam before the gin-shop, so dense that nothing can disturb it, except the tawdry bacchantes blundering about the pavement to its music. I am not an ultramoralist. I have been long enough fighting the battles of life upon town, to stand a great deal that is very equivocal, unflinchingly: but I do say, that this corner of the Haymarket is a cancer in the great heart of the Metropolis, and a shame and a disgrace to the supervision of any police. A convivial 'drunky', who inclines to harmony as he goes home at night, when there is not a soul in his way to be annoyed, by expressing his confidence, through all changes, in dog Tray's fidelity, has been quieted, before this, by a knock on the head from a truncheon. A poor apple-woman, striving to earn a wretched pittance against the birth of an infant evidently not far off, is chased from post to pillar by any numbered letter of the alphabet; but here, wanton wickedness riots unchecked. The edge of the pavement is completely blockaded. If you happen to be accompanied by wife, daughter, sister, any decent woman, and to be waiting, or not waiting for one of the omnibuses that must pass there – go anywhere, do anything, rather than attempt to elbow through the phalanx of rogues, and thieves, and nameless shames and horrors.

From an extensive continental experience of cities, I can take personally an example from three-quarters of the globe; but I have never anywhere witnessed such open ruffianism and wretched profligacy as rings along those Piccadilly flagstones any time after the gas is lighted.

It is during the weeks of Epsom, Ascot, and Hampton, that the disciples of Thurtell's school of pursuits hold high festival.[53] Two or three years back, there were various betting houses here, with their traps always set open to catch their prey; but although these are abolished, something of the kind is still going on, which the police know (or pretend to know) nothing about. The swarm of low sporting ruffians hovering about here, at all times, is incredible. You know they have all figured, are figuring, or will figure, in card-cheating cases and dirty bill transactions. They have all the bandy legs and tight trousers, the freckled faces and speckled hands, and grubby, dubby nails that distinguish this fraternity. Theirs are the strong-flavoured cigar and highly-coloured brandy, the snaffle coat-links, and large breast-pin, the vulgar stock, and the hat-band – always the hat-band; is it a last clinging to respectability, to show that there was somebody belonging to them once? And when to this unsavoury locust-cloud the closing casino adds its different but equally obstructive swarm, and they all flutter about in the lamp-lights, amidst an admiring audience of pickpockets, flower-sellers, rich country fools, who think they are 'seeing life', and poor scamps who show it to them, such a witch's cauldron is seething in the public eye, and splashing in the face of decency, as is quite intolerable to this land at this date.

I entreat the intelligent magistrates in whose division ROGUES' WALK lies, to leave their dinner-tables some evening, and go and judge for themselves whether it is anybody's business to do anything towards the correction of this scene of profligacy. Why should no quiet person be able to walk upon its skirts, unmolested, and why should all modest ears and eyes be shocked and outraged in one of the greatest thoroughfares of this Metropolis?

APPENDIX B

THE ARGYLL ROOMS IN THE EIGHTEEN-FIFTIES

The following is a shortened version of the article in the Saturday Review, *October 16, 1853, quoted in full by Acton in a footnote (see p. 163).*

Public decency is in a difficulty, and it seems that the remedy is worse than the disease. We appear to be in that condition which the Roman historian has described as the vice of a falling State – we can neither endure our vices nor their cures. Last year, in a transport of moral and popular indignation, we closed the Argyll Rooms because they were the focus and complex of all metropolitan vice. This year we open them, because, on the whole, it is better that the vicious population should be brought together than that it should be let loose on society. There is antecedently much to be said for either view of the moral question. A whole cloud of evidence was brought, on the recent occasion of the proprietor of the Rooms applying for a licence, to show that the streets have been in a worse state since the lorettes of London were deprived of their customary home, than when they had a local habitation. And, had the evidence stopped here, it might have proved something. But, unfortunately, the proprietor went beyond this. The justification of such an institution is that it is a moral cesspool. But it cannot be at the same time a cesspool and a healing fountain. Evidence was tendered that the Argyll Rooms were frequented by respectable tradesmen and their wives. Five or six hundred noblemen and gentlemen are said to have offered, or to have been ready to offer, their testimony to the admirable way in which the Rooms were conducted. The music is of the most scientific character, order and decorum find their chosen home in Windmill Street, and the evidence at least suggests that casinos divide with the pulpit the duty of preserving the general social health of London. This is proving a little too much. Had the argument confined itself to the one simple ground that immorality must be, and that on the whole it is better that immorality and its haunts should be under decent and responsible management and control, we own to a growing conviction that it was right to grant the licence – not because the

Argyll Rooms are a moral institution, but because, so long as they are open under the care and responsibility of a respectable, or at least substantial person, public morality suffers less than when harlotry unattached turns a whole quarter of London to an unlicensed Argyll Rooms and something worse.

The Argyll Rooms, and casinos generally, are known to be the haunts of the *femmes libres* of society. This is, if fairly stated, their justification. The objection urged to licensing them is that we do evil that good may ensue – that we openly recognize, and so far authenticate and stamp with the authority of the State and Government, a flagrant violation of the moral law. It is said that we establish, and so far encourage, immorality as soon as we recognize it. . . . Has the State moral duties or not? If it has, if it is bound to provide for public decency, it must, in the grave matter of sexual immorality, do one of two things – either attempt utterly to prohibit sins against the seventh commandment, and to enforce the prohibition, or so far tolerate them as at least to admit their existence by dealing with them. To talk of prohibiting prostitution and the like is absurd. What there is left for the State is to deal with this and other social evils so as to render them less generally noxious. By dishonestly affecting to deny their existence, we commit an offence not only against truth but against policy. . . . Public morality is more confined in its range than individual duty. It acts upon motives necessarily less heroic – it cannot be so severe and austere in its consistency. If it cannot prohibit prostitution, its first duty is to make the best of it. We have made the worst of it by the impolicy of affecting not to see it.

If, therefore, we are to accept the licensing of the Argyll Rooms as a public recognition of vice to the extent of placing it under public control, and as a step, not to the system of licensing immoral houses as on the Continent, but to the public and authoritative control of immorality, we should be disposed to accept with some satisfaction the decision of the Middlesex magistrates. What can't be cured must be alleviated. . . . It is better that some hundred females of loose life should be entertained for a few hours in a single room, than that they should be encouraged to prowl about the streets. Whatever thins the loose population of the Haymarket and Regent Street is so far a social gain. We ought to regard the interests, not of the profligate, but of the respectable. At all events, when vice is concentrated in Windmill Street, men must go in cold blood to seek it out, while, flaunting on the *pavé*, it tempts the young and unwary. Few except extreme profligates would go to the recognized haunts of vice; but many fall under the public temptation of the streets who would avoid it in its own dancing and drinking saloons.

At any rate, the lesson taught by the change of opinion on the part of the Middlesex magistrates since last year is, that it will not do to attempt a system of prosecuting these vicious places by instalments. There is already power in the common law to hunt down immorality by units and in detail. All immoral houses can be suppressed by the parochial authorities – all street-walkers may be arrested by the police. But to carry out the law is simply impossible. What is cut down in one street grows up in the next – the weeds are only transported from Norton Street to Brompton. It is of no use to prohibit – all that we can do is to regulate. We had rather not see a parochial crusade against immorality, for the evil will only be transferred to the other side of the boundary. Let authority deal with any offence against public decency; let the magistrate, or the police, receive additional powers to repress public offences; but the failure of the attempt to put down the Argyll Rooms shows that we are beginning to understand that to control is better than an abortive attempt to prohibit.

APPENDIX C

MANNERS AND MORALS OF STOCKHOLM

This extract from Northern Travel (*1858*), *by Bayard Taylor,*[54] *is another of Acton's footnotes, in the chapter on 'Prostitution Abroad'. It is taken from p. 189 of Taylor's book.*

It has been called the most licentious city in Europe, and, I have no doubt, with the most perfect justice. Vienna may surpass it in the amount of conjugal infidelity, but certainly not in general incontinence. Very nearly half the registered births are illegitimate, to say nothing of the illegitimate children born *in* wedlock. Of the servant girls, shop girls, and seamstresses in the city, it is very safe to say that scarcely ten out of a hundred are chaste, while, as rakish young Swedes have coolly informed me, many girls of respectable parentage, belonging to the middle-class, are not much better. The men, of course, are much worse than the women, and even in Paris one sees fewer physical signs of excessive debauchery. Here the number of broken-down young men, and blear-eyed, hoary sinners, is astonishing. I have never been in any place where licentiousness was so open and avowed – and yet, where the slang of a sham morality was so prevalent. There are no houses of prostitution in Stockholm, and the city would be scandalized at the idea of allowing such a thing. A few years ago two were established, and the fact was no sooner known than a virtuous mob arose and violently pulled them down! At the restaurants, young blades order their dinners of the female waiters with an arm around their waists, while the old men place their hands unblushingly upon their bosoms. All the baths in Stockholm are attended by women (generally middle-aged and hideous, I must confess), who perform the usual scrubbing and shampoo-ing with the greatest nonchalance. One does not wonder when he is told of young men who have passed safely through the ordeals of Berlin and Paris, and have come at last to Stockholm to be ruined.

APPENDIX D

TWO REVIEWS OF ACTON'S
PROSTITUTION

The following is a shortened version of the notice (of the first edition) in the
Sanitary Review and Journal of Public Health, *III (1857–58), 327–35.*

THE SOCIAL EPIDEMIC

The subject of the work in hand has been so freely discussed in the
periodicals of the day, that it would be mere prudery to offer any apology
for drawing attention to its contents. No one at all acquainted with the
state of modern society will be at all disposed to deny that the evil of
which the book treats is of immense magnitude, for its roots extend deep
into the soil on which our present social fabric rests, whilst its branches
overshadow the privacies of our domestic life. It is an evil which leaves
its traces discoverable by the eye of the physician among all classes of the
people, and from which neither riches form a safeguard nor poverty a
protection.

It is an ungracious task to hold up the mirror and show the form and
pressure of the time; for, while it shows us our railways, telegraphs, and
leviathan steamers, our monster meetings for preachings, for social
science, and for the fine arts, it shows us withal a shady side of vice and
sensuality, which in magnitude can only be likened to that of the accursed
cities of antiquity. We sing an everlasting 'Io Pæan' on progress, on the
march of intellect, and on national prosperity. We plume ourselves on
subjugating the elements, we overcome the winds and the waves, and try
to annihilate time and space. Now and then, with great timidity, some
chivalrous man of science ventures gently to raise the veil . . . which
screens our social habits, and gives us a view of the obscene mysteries,
which are being constantly enacted in our streets, and a picture of
manners comparable only with the wildest saturnalia of the worst of
pagan times. In the book before us, we have the death's head and cross
bones brought into the feasts of good society; and enough is related to mar
the complacency of the most well-bred conventionalist.

Whoever knows anything of London life, will at once confess that the evil which the author has endeavoured to describe he has not at all attempted to exaggerate. The actual misery and disease need no description. They describe themselves, and may be seen in the streets, unless kept out of sight by the police. Those who require facts and figures for conviction, must read the statistics of venereal diseases. The author marshals his facts which look like a funeral procession; he preaches a funeral oration on the death of national chastity. He does more; he gives us a *post mortem* examination, and demonstrates that our seeming virtue is little other than a whited sepulchre.... In treating of the causes of prostitution, the author frequently quotes Mr Mayhew's letters to the *Morning Chronicle*, in which the demoralization of children is described as taking place in the low lodging-houses of London and elsewhere. It will suffice to say, that these letters describe scenes of juvenile precocity in vice, which the narrator confesses cannot be detailed in print....

It can hardly excite surprise that a sort of practical communism should prevail among the lower orders. The value of chastity is not appreciated by them as it should be.... It would appear that we are 'drifting' into a sea of socialism. As to the extent to which prostitution prevails, it is impossible to form any approximative calculation.

It can easily be understood that this is a profession which, whether it be practised for love or money, is usually carried on as privately as possible, and that it is only the open and avowed courtesans who are constantly walking the streets, or who inhabit houses of ill-fame, that are likely to come under the cognizance of the authorities. But this class forms but an insignificant portion of the female community who are living in more or less open concubinage. As the wages accorded to female labour in slopwork, millinery, dressmaking, bookbinding, artificial flower making, etc., are not such as to afford an honest subsistence, many girls who have not other means beside their work are partly compelled by want, partly encouraged by example, and partly tempted by pleasure, to leave the steep and thorny way to heaven, for the primrose path of dalliance.

It would appear almost a work of supererogation to quote figures to prove that prostitution prevails to an enormous extent; however, those exquisite optimists who desire to learn the truth would do well to look into Mr Acton's book, where they will find the evidence of all classes. The clergy, the police, the reputable householders and municipal corporations, the medical men and hospitals, all testify to the extent of the moral disease. We shall therefore take it as an established fact, that all the accounts we hear are not exaggerated.

The only excuse for bringing this subject before the eye of the general public, is the hope that reformation may be brought about. The publication of the details of a revolting traffic; the natural history of the professed woman of the streets; the description of the means and appliances of professed bawds and their modes of communication with their patrons, is not an unmixed good to the community. Although a scientific investigator may be called upon to detail the results of his experience, and although the *littérateur* may find his end in giving photographic representations of filth and low debauchery, and although this may stimulate the really good to exert themselves for the amelioration of vice, yet, to the sensual, the vicious, the young and inexperienced, these scientific books thus popularized are too liable to be converted into mere guide-books to vice, or to afford amusement to the prurient fancy of the depraved; and thus, as it were, they hold a candle to the devil, by suggesting means and appliances for vicious indulgences which otherwise might never have been thought of. . . .

We cannot follow Mr Acton in his *Harlot's Progress*, nor accompany him in his peregrinations through their *Homes and Haunts of London*; through *dress-houses*; houses in which prostitutes lodge; introducing houses; accommodation houses; casinos; pleasure gardens; and the streets. But we proceed to the consideration whether any means can be suggested for the mitigation of the evil. First, it may be asked, whether legislation can do any good. There is great doubt whether good can come of endeavouring to make people virtuous by acts of parliament. . . . We dare not go so far as the hope of Mr Acton, that the day may come when the communication of syphilis to a minor may be made a felony. . . . Nor is it so clear that all the centralization of despotic bureaucracy is a match for the spread of licentiousness. If we are to believe all accounts of the doings in Paris, in Naples, in Madrid, and in nearly all the capitals of Europe, we shall have to bewail more over the degeneracy of morals in general, than of London in particular. And if we compare the prevalence of venereal disease in military hospitals of different countries, we find that notwithstanding all police and medical arrangements, our *laisser aller* system, as it is called, is not so prejudicial as might have been expected. . . .

It does seem that the only practical way of doing any good to the unfortunate who may be suffering from this disease, would be to increase the hospital and dispensary accommodation for this especial complaint, and to let it be on the same principle as that of the Royal Free Hospital. Start a hospital or dispensary for all comers, and let there be no historical questions asked of the miserable sufferers; let disease be the simple letter of recommendation, and then, no doubt, the sick will avail themselves of such a charity with heartfelt gratitude. No one likes to publish his own disgrace: then why should we expect that women should prove an exception? Nay, rather, we think, would they suffer disease and death, than let all the world know their degradation. We cannot therefore hope, nor indeed could we wish, that Englishwomen, however low they may have descended in their habits, would yet voluntarily enrol themselves either as professional prostitutes, or as members of a prostitutes' mutual aid and sanitary society.

Whether from the increasing decay of morals, or whether from the publicity now given by the press to all the vices of the age, it is certain that great uneasiness is felt by all thinking people at the progress which vice seems to be making amongst us; and people are naturally anxious, if only for self-preservation, that some check should be placed on its development. Neither laws nor punishments can ever supply the place of sound moral training; and all the centralization in the world will never reform an iniquitous age. Concubinage, which is but a substitute for polygamy, is generally considered as a token of national decline.

There is an evil, possibly even greater than that which has been called the greatest of our social evils; and that is, the consummate class selfishness which prevails. This feeling recognizes only the elect, and abandons the rest to reprobation. *Respectability* is the name under which this principle is personified and worshipped. Her votaries live within a charmed circle, comfortably supplied with everything requisite for their physical and spiritual wants. They have good tables, and soft seats in the place of worship. Well dressed, well gloved, and well scented, they carry prayer-books bound in curious antique; they behave decorously, make all responses, and sing *sotto voce*. Well may they congratulate themselves! The votary of *Disreputability* acknowledges that her goddess has a brazen impudent carriage, but says she is no more than what she professes to be, whilst she accuses Respectability of being little better than a solemn mockery. Open blackguardism is what she prefers, rather than organized and conventional hypocrisy.

We must conclude this notice of Mr Acton's book, and pay a tribute to his courage in bringing before the British public the dark side of their social condition. It must evidently tend to ameliorate this state of things. What are Church and State about, that they take no heed of the times? Have they adopted the motto, *Après moi le déluge*? We shall see.

The second edition was noticed as follows in the Lancet, *1870, I. 161–2.*

Mr Acton has improved his work on Prostitution in this second edition; it is, on the whole, a good exposition of an evil that in many ways is working both physical and moral harm to all classes of society, but probably even more so in the latter than in the former respect. The work discusses ... the causes, amelioration, and prevention by regulation of prostitution in general, and especially of prostitution in the Metropolis. The diseases that result from prostitution, and the means in London for curing them, are compared with the same conditions in certain foreign cities, much to the advantage of the latter. The extent of prostitution is very imperfectly known, and Mr Acton has rendered a service by discussing the subject, and furnishing us with an account of the evil. It is, nevertheless, to be regretted that the author should have allowed himself to introduce sensational matter into his history of a most repulsive subject; letters from Belgravian mothers and their respondents, culled from the *Daily Telegraph* and *The Times*, were quite unnecessary. Still more objectionable are highly coloured autobiographies of women of loose character, or picturesque descriptions of evenings spent at Cremorne and elsewhere.

It is pointed out with some force how much of the demand for prostitution is due to lads and young men not being properly trained. Prostitution is also fostered by the artificial impediment that modern society throws in the way of early marriages, with which may be included the unwillingness of many to assume the obligations of married life. These, the chief sources of *demand*, are stimuli to others guiding the *supply* – namely, dislike of honest labour, and vicious inclinations inculcated by evil training and by the indecent crowding together that so many thousands of our lower classes cannot avoid. To these may be added the difficulty in obtaining employment that compels fallen women to resort to prostitution for a subsistence, the pinching of extreme poverty, the love of dress, domestic unhappiness, and the exposure to temptation that especially assails domestic servants. Both demand and supply are also subject to a fictitious stimulation of various kinds, which we hold the State should endeavour to remove, or reduce as much as possible; but this cannot be done by ignoring what is well known to exist by everyone. A prohibition of prostitution has never been attended with success. This has been attempted at various epochs in Berlin, but on each occasion the result of repression has been to increase the number of illegitimate births, of infanticides, and of venereal patients. Between 1845 and 1848, the last time that prohibition has been attempted in Berlin, the entries at the hospital for syphilis rose from 711 to 979. In the Papal States prostitution has been repressed; but, as far as Rome is concerned, this has only served to develop new and worse evils. Some people talk as if advance in morals were strictly comparable to mental progress. Every accession to knowledge in one age necessarily affects the intellectual progress of the next; but animalism and the temptations to vice repeat themselves; their external manifestations may and do change, but their nature does not. Mr Acton has obtained some official information, with the help of our Government, respecting the management of prostitution at Berlin, in which it is stated that the entries for venereal in the Prussian Army were only 62 per 1,000 in 1867, against 258 in our own army.

We must dispute Mr Acton's inference respecting the number of prostitutes in London. No precise expression of opinion on this point is given, but he leads us to suppose the number to be enormous. At present we are inclined to think we might take the police estimate as the number with which a Contagious Diseases Act could deal at first; and this will enable us to arrive at a fair estimate of the amount of money we are likely to require to effect a sensible diminution of venereal disease. Each bed at the London Lock Hospital costs £24 10s. per year, and accommodates about eleven patients annually. Now of the 6,000 common prostitutes, about one-third, or at most one-half, are diseased, and would require an immediate accommodation of 3,000 beds. This is probably more than could be granted; and if we turn to the statistics of Berlin, we find that 120 women are generally in hospital, out of 1,600; say 160 – i.e., 10 per cent; or 600 beds are the proportion that would be necessary as a permanent provision for the 6,000 common prostitutes of London. With this accommodation we should provide for the treatment of all the diseased *most common* women; and so cut off communication with all the worst and most multiplying seed-beds of disease. As the value of the measure became more apparent, there would be less difficulty in obtaining funds for ampler accommodation.

In estimating the amount of sickness disseminated by prostitution, Mr Acton so states his case as to mislead respecting the number of hospital venereal patients. The error lies in not mentioning that the statistics Mr Acton collected referred only to the surgical out-patients, and did not include the medical out-patients also, who, as every hospital officer knows, far outnumber the surgical patients. This oversight is fatal to his statistics, and is especially damaging, since it has been opposed by data collected by Mr Simon. Without allowing that Mr Simon's estimate is correct, probably it is as far below the mark as Mr Acton's in its present form is above the real quantity; we regret it did not occur to Mr Acton to weigh Mr Simon's statements against his own, when treating of the prevalence of venereal disease. Another source of fallacy is this: the tables of the mortality from syphilis in the Registrar-General's report, and in the venereal wards of certain hospitals, are inserted without any explanation to show whether Mr Acton is aware that these official returns give but a part of the true mortality from syphilis, and that many deaths from disease set in action by syphilis are described as due to affections of other organs.

In the chapter on the Amelioration of Prostitution, Mr Acton has grappled with the objections in the Report of the Medical Officer of the Privy Council to the extension of the Contagious Diseases Act to the civil population. *Imprimis*: in answer to Mr Simon's assertion that the principle at stake in the proposed alteration is 'whether the venereal diseases of the civil population are henceforth to be deemed matter of public concern, whether the civil fornicant may reasonably look to constituted authorities to protect him in his commerce with prostitutes?' – Mr Acton expresses his well-founded amazement that Mr Simon should for a moment suppose these two definitions of the principle at stake to be synonymous. Such a confusion of ideas (and Mr Simon's argument is based throughout on this confusion) naturally deprives Mr Simon's judgment of the question of the weight that utterances of his ought to command. Mr Acton cleverly shows how exactly contrary is the opinion that Mr Simon expresses concerning the right – and even the duty – of the law to intervene and limit the liberty of the subject in order to prevent the spread of disease when he quits the topic of venereal affections. By turning to the next page of Mr Simon's Report we find him saying that 'it is the almost completely expressed intention of our law that all such states of property and all such modes of personal action or inaction, as may be of danger to the public health, should be brought within the scope of summary procedure and conviction', with much more to the same purpose, showing Mr Simon to be guilty of strange inconsistency when deliberating on the duty of the State in regard of venereal and other sources of preventable disease.

NOTES

1. The Contagious Diseases Acts, 1864, 1866, and 1869, were passed to prevent venereal diseases by the medical examination of prostitutes and the detention in hospital of those found to be diseased. The 1864 Act applied to the garrison towns of Portsmouth, Plymouth, Woolwich, Chatham, Sheerness, Aldershot, Colchester, Shorncliffe, The Curragh, Cork, and Queenstown. It provided that, within these areas, a police superintendent or inspector could lay information before a justice of the peace that he had reason to believe a certain woman was a common prostitute. The J.P. could then order the woman to be medically examined and – if she were found to be suffering from a venereal disease – detained in hospital for treatment for a period of up to three months. If the woman did not wish to appear in court, she could sign a voluntary submission. By the 1866 Act a J.P. could order a woman informed against as a common prostitute to undergo periodical medical examination for a year. The maximum period of hospital detention was increased to six months, and Windsor was added to the scheduled areas. The 1869 Act increased the maximum detention in hospital to nine months and added Canterbury, Dover, Gravesend, Maidstone, Winchester, and Southampton to the scheduled areas.

A National Association for Repeal and a Ladies' National Association for Repeal were formed, and in 1869 the latter issued a manifesto signed by 124 women, including Florence Nightingale (1820–1910) and Josephine Butler (1828–1906), who became leader of the movement against the Acts. The agitation led to the appointment in 1879 of a Select Committee, which reported three years later. The majority was in favour of the Acts' continuing. But a minority report, signed by six members – including Sir James Stansfeld (1820–98), former financial secretary to the Treasury – held that venereal diseases in the home army had not been reduced; that they had increased among registered women; that the only good done by police employed under the Acts was beyond their duties and would be better done by other means; and that there was merit in the religious, moral, and constitutional objections to the Acts. They were suspended in 1883 and repealed in 1886.

2. The Foundling Hospital, established in 1739 by Captain Thomas Coram (c. 1668–1751) 'for the maintenance and education of exposed and deserted young children', moved to Lamb's Conduit Fields in 1754.

See R. H. Nichols and F. A. Wray, *The History of the Foundling Hospital* (1935). It survives today as the Thomas Coram Foundation for Children.

3. Edward Henry Stanley (1826–93), 15th earl of Derby, was secretary of state for foreign affairs, 1866–68 and 1874–78.

4. William Farr (1807–83) was a leading authority on medical and public health statistics.

5. Captain William Charles Harris (1809–87) was chief constable of Hampshire, 1843–56, and assistant commissioner of the Metropolitan Police, 1856–81. He wrote *Questions and Answers Framed for the Instruction of Constables on Joining the Police* (1860) and *A Manual of Drill, Prepared for the Use of the County and District Constables* (1862).

6. The Hon. John Cranch Walker Vivian (1818–79), captain in the 11th Hussars, was M.P. for Truro and elsewhere, and at various times lord of the Treasury and permanent under-secretary to the War Office.

7. William Henry Sloggett (d. 1887?), Member of the Royal College of Surgeons, 1841, was awarded the Gilbert Blane medal in 1866 and served as deputy inspector general of hospitals and fleets, 1874–75.

8. Sir John Somerset Pakington (1799–1880) was twice secretary for war and twice first lord of the Admiralty. In 1867 he indiscreetly revealed the secret history of the Reform Bill (the 'Ten Minutes Bill'). He was created baron Hampton in 1874.

9. William Brewer (d. 1881), M.P. for Colchester, 1868–74, wrote *The Family Medical Reference Book* (1840) and an historical novel, *Beatrice Sforza or, the Progress of Truth* (1863).

10. Edward Kent Parsons (1820–90) was on the staff of the Royal Portsmouth Hospital for thirty-five years, till his retirement in 1885. He was a magistrate for Portsmouth.

11. John Simon (1816–1904) was medical officer to the Privy Council, 1855–76, and author of *English Sanitary Institutions* (1890). He was knighted in 1887.

12. Patrick Colquhoun (1745–1820), metropolitan police magistrate, 1792–1818, wrote *Suggestions . . . with a View to the Encouragement of Soup Establishments* (1798) and many other works. His *Treatise on the Police of the Metropolis* was first published, anonymously, in 1796, and his estimate of the number of prostitutes in London appeared in the fifth edition (1797), 421 n. No basis was given for the calculation, on which the *London City Mission Magazine*, V (1840), 166, commented: 'It is well known that many of his calculations were singularly inaccurate.' Cf. *Foreign Quarterly Review*, XIX (1837), 340, where Colquhoun's *Treatise*

234

234

is described as 'a work possessing more authority than it has any title to claim'.

13. Henry Phillpotts (1778–1869) was bishop of Exeter from 1830 to his death. A high churchman, he defended the Peterloo massacre (1819) and the Poor Law, opposed Catholic emancipation and the Reform Bill, and had protracted ecclesiastical lawsuits with several of the clergy in his diocese on questions of discipline, patronage, and heresy.

14. James Beard Talbot (1800 or 1801–1881), author of *The Miseries of Prostitution* (1844), was secretary of the London Society for the Protection of Young Females and Prevention of Juvenile Prostitution, which he founded at Tottenham in 1835. It later moved to Woodhouse, Wanstead, and the name was changed to the Princess Louise Home. Acton takes Talbot's estimate (and, it seems, Colquhoun's), without acknowledgment, from Michael Ryan, *Prostitution in London* (1839), 168, 89.

15. Sir Richard Mayne (1796–1868), a barrister, was joint commissioner of the Metropolitan Police from 1829, chief commissioner from 1850.

16. John Smith was inspector of the Metropolitan Police at Aldershot for the purposes of the Contagious Diseases Act, 1866. His duties consisted in watching for women who were supposed to be prostitutes, warning them to attend for medical examination, and conveying them to and from the hospital.

17. John Coleman Barr (d. 1899?), formerly resident medical officer at the Female Lock Hospital, Harrow Road, London, was medical officer at the Aldershot Lock Hospital and visiting medical officer for the district under the Contagious Diseases Acts.

18. *lupanaria*, brothels. From Latin *lupa*, she-wolf, whore.

19. *over the water,* south of the Thames.

20. Cremorne Gardens, a 12-acre (later 16-acre) site off the King's Road, Chelsea, were first opened in 1830 by 'baron' Charles Random de Berenger, for sports, galas, *fêtes-champêtres*, balloon ascents, fireworks, music, and dancing, and were revived in 1843 by Renton Nicholson, the self-styled 'lord chief baron'. After long opposition to their licence by the Chelsea Vestry and the Chelsea Baptists, the gardens were closed in 1877. See Warwick Wroth, *Cremorne and the Later London Gardens* (1907). Acton's description of Cremorne may be compared with J. Ewing Ritchie's, in *The Night Side of London* (1857), 183–91.

21. *Terpsichore*, the muse of dancing. *Melpomene*, the muse of tragedy.

22. *etiolated*, blanched. *chlorotic*, affected with chlorosis, or green

sickness. *defibrinization*, deprival of fibrin, the protein which forms the essential part of the blood clot.

23. The gardens attached to the Pavilion Hotel, north Woolwich, were open from 1851 to *c.* 1883. Highbury Barn gardens, from *c.* 1830, were a kind of north London Cremorne; having lost their dancing licence because of neighbours' complaints of riotous behaviour, they were closed in 1871. Highbury Barn in the 1850s is described in J. Ewing Ritchie, *The Night Side of London* (1857), 152–7. The Rosherville gardens, laid out in a chalk pit between Gravesend and Northfleet, were opened in 1837 and closed in 1920.

24. The notorious Argyll Rooms in Great Windmill Street were opened, between 1849 and 1851, by a wine merchant named Robert Bignell, who made a large fortune out of them. The author of *My Secret Life* describes them as 'the resort of the handsomest and best-dressed gay women' (IV. 199; Grove Press edition, I. 750); H. G. Hibbert, in *A Playgoer's Memories* (1920), 250–1, compared them to 'a modern night club, without its perfunctory condition of election to membership. You just bought a ticket and went in – to mix with the *demi-reps* and the *demi-mondaines* who danced and drank till morning'. Bignell was ultimately deprived of his music and dancing licence, and the Argyll Rooms closed in 1878, police preventing a 'lusty last night' by forming a cordon round Windmill Street and driving back the 'angry roisterers'. Bignell reopened the premises four years later as a music hall called the Trocadero Palace, which was acquired by J. Lyons and Co. Ltd in 1895 and turned into a restaurant. For an 1853 reference to the Argyll Rooms, see Appendix B, pp. 221–3 above.

The National Assembly Rooms (formerly Casino de Venise or Holborn Casino) at 218 High Holborn was a similar dancing-place. It closed down in 1872 as a consequence of that year's Licensing Act, which fixed midnight as the closing hour for premises supplying intoxicating drinks within four miles of Charing Cross.

25. *Ratcliff Highway in 1842*, a song celebrating 'all the most famous public houses in and about that famous street, and the ladies who frequented them', will be found in Millicent Rose, *The East End of London* (1951), 220–1. The author of *My Secret Life*, 'dressed in the shabbiest possible manner', visited what was probably the Ratcliffe Highway area in the late 1850s (VI. 289–97; Grove Press edition, I. 1239–43); his description may be compared with that in J. Ewing Ritchie, *The Night Side of London* (1857), 66–75.

26. The Alhambra, in Leicester Square, was opened in 1858, and became famous, from 1864, for its spectacular ballets and the promenade to which unescorted women were admitted.

27. For 'Blackwall parties', see Millicent Rose, *The East End of London* (1951), 150: 'On summer evenings in the forties Blackwall was a favourite resort for excursionists from the City. At the old public houses along the river, whitebait suppers could be eaten in a marine setting, a combination much to the taste of the times.'

28. Major George Graham (1801–88) was military secretary at Bombay, 1828–30, and registrar-general of births, marriages, and deaths, 1838–79.

29. *phagedaenic disease*, rapidly spreading and sloughing ulceration. The term *phagedaena* is used by Acton to indicate a form of chancre.

30. *cachexia*, general ill health and malnutrition.

31. *rupia*, a skin disease.

32. Exeter Hall, in the Strand, was built in 1831 and used for the annual meetings of religious societies and for the oratorios performed by the Sacred Harmonic Society. In 1880 it was taken over, and partly rebuilt, by the Young Men's Christian Association. The hall was demolished in 1907.

33. John Wilson (1788–1870) compiled the earliest volumes of naval medical statistics, wrote *Medical Notes on the War in China* (1846), and was inspector of Greenwich Hospital, 1855–61.

34. George Busk (1807–86) was surgeon to the Seamen's Hospital during the early part of his career, Hunterian professor of comparative anatomy and physiology, 1856–59, author of zoological and anthropological papers, and translator of standard works on histology.

35. Sir Astley Paston Cooper, Bt (1768–1841), the leading surgeon of his time, was one of the founders of the Medico-Chirurgical Society (1805) and author of works on hernia (1804–7), the testis (1830), the thymus gland (1832), and the anatomy of the breast (1840), as well as *Lectures ... on the Principles and Practice of Surgery*, ed. Frederick Tyrrell (1824–27). There are biographies by his nephew, B. B. Cooper (1843), Geoffrey Keynes (1922), and Russell C. Brock (1952). The passage referred to by Acton occurs in Cooper's *Lectures*, second edition (1830), 515.

For phagedaena, see note 29 above. Acton told the Lords Committee on the Contagious Diseases Act, 1866: 'In the Peninsular War there was a complaint called the black lion of Portugal, resulting from the soldiers being diseased, and drinking new wine; under these unfavourable sanitary arrangements the penis sloughed off' (*Report from the Select Committee of the House of Lords on the Contagious Diseases Act, 1866* (1868), q. 924).

36. *spermatorrhoea*, a pseudo-disease invented by Claude-François Lallemand (1790–1854), a French professor of clinical surgery and author of *Des pertes séminales involontaires* (Paris and Montpellier, 1836–42). The symptoms included wet dreams, loss of semen while defecating, imperfect or transient erections, premature ejaculation, watery semen, imperceptible loss of semen with the urine, and impotence. Almost the entire medical profession, throughout the second half of the nineteenth century, believed that masturbation led to 'spermatorrhoea', and a work on the subject by John Laws Milton (1820–98), a lecturer on diseases of the skin, went through twelve editions in little more than thirty years. It grew with each recension, so that what started as a fourteen-page pamphlet reprinted from the *Lancet* (1854, I. 243–6, 269–70, 467–8, 595–6) had become a 213-page book by 1887. In this book of Milton's will be found details of the electric alarum and the urethral ring. The former consisted of a ring placed on the penis at night; expanded by erection, it completed an electric current, so ringing a small alarm bell under the sleeper's pillow. (Contrary to general belief, this seems not to have been a device to make fathers aware of their sons' nocturnal erections; as Milton describes it, the object was to prevent nocturnal emissions in adults.) The urethral ring, manufactured by F. Walters and Co., of Moorgate Street, London, came in two varieties, four-pointed and toothed. The former was made of leather. Tied on the penis with a little bow, it opened out and pricked the sleeper as soon as erection occurred. If the patient found himself beginning to untie the ring in his sleep, he was advised to substitute for the tape securing it a hook and eye and small padlock – and to place the key out of reach. The toothed urethral ring, made of a very thin watch-spring covered with silk, operated similarly.

37. James Robert Lane (1825–91) was consulting surgeon to St Mary's Hospital, London, till 1881. His 1876 Harveian lectures were published as *Lectures on Syphilis* (1878).

38. George Frederick Samuel Robinson (1827–1909), 3rd earl De Grey and 2nd earl (afterwards 1st marquess) of Ripon, was secretary of state for war, 1863–66, lord president of the council, 1868–73, and viceroy of India, 1880–84.

39. William Reginald Courtenay (1807–88), 11th earl of Devon, a

barrister, was secretary to the Poor Law Board, 1850–59, and president, 1867–68.

40. William Wells Addington (1824–1913), 3rd viscount Sidmouth, was M.P. for Devizes, 1863–64.

41. Edward Gordon Douglas-Pennant (1800–86), 1st baron Penrhyn, was M.P. for Carnarvonshire, 1841–66.

42. George Frederick Uptown (1802–90), 3rd viscount Templetown, a general, was M.P. for Antrim, 1859–63.

43. Kate Hamilton's, Rose Young's, and Coney's were celebrated 'night houses' of the 1860s. Coney's was frequented by sporting men. Kate Hamilton's, smartest and most popular of such places, is thus described by Ralph Nevill, *Night Life: London and Paris – Past and Present* (1926), 38–9: 'After a certain hour at night the proprietress was always to be found seated on a sort of throne placed on a raised platform, from which she was wont to greet visitors of note. Weighing some twenty stone, with a countenance which had weathered countless convivial nights, Mrs Hamilton presented a stupendous appearance in the low-cut evening dresses which she always wore. From midnight to dawn she sipped champagne, sharing bottles with young men about town, who regarded an invitation to sit by the presiding goddess of the place as a privilege likely to enhance their prestige with the soiled doves who were then more gently treated than is the case today. Kate Hamilton, with her foghorn voice, knew how to keep her clients of both sexes in order, and on the whole her establishment seems not to have been any more noxious than the dancing-places which exist in Montmartre today. The amusements to be found there, indeed, seem generally to have been more decorous than those to be procured in modern Parisian night resorts. No semi-nude dancing prevailed, while the supper consisted of cold beef and other simple English dishes, washed down, it is true, by copious draughts of champagne. Occasionally there was a row, and in latter days a raid. However, long before the police had come in, bottles and glasses had been concealed much as they are in the illicit night clubs of today. In private life Kate Hamilton was a respected member of the congregation of a well-known church, and figured in the Court Guide as occupying a house in a good street.'

44. By 'the street connecting Leicester Square with the bottom of Regent Street', Acton appears to mean Coventry Street.

45. Sir Peter Laurie (1779?–1861), lord mayor of London, 1832, wrote pamphlets (1846, 1848) on prison reform.

46. See note 11 above.

47. The Association for Promoting the Extension of the Contagious Diseases Act, 1866, to the Civil Population of the United Kingdom, had in 1868 a membership of about 400, including about thirty M.P.s and two bishops. Its first secretary was the venereologist Dr Berkeley Hill (1834–92).

48. The Hon. Baptist Wriothesley Noel (1798–1873), minister of John Street Baptist Chapel, London, 1849–68, was a highly popular preacher and author of many tracts and several travel books.

49. Edward Henry Bickersteth (1825–1906) was vicar of Christ Church, Hampstead, 1855–85, and bishop of Exeter, 1885–1900. He wrote religious prose and verse, including 'Peace, Perfect Peace' (1883) and other hymns.

50. William Brock (1807–75) was pastor of Bloomsbury Chapel, London, 1848–72, one of the founders of the London Association of Baptist Churches, and president of the Baptist Union, 1869. He wrote *The Midsummer Morning Sermons to Young Men and Maidens* [1872] and numerous other works. There are biographies by George W. MacCree (1876) and Charles M. Birrell (1878).

51. *marasmus*, progressive wasting and emaciation, especially in infants.

52. Albert Richard Smith (1816–60) was a well-known author, lecturer, and public entertainer. His novels include *The Adventures of Mr Ledbury and his Friend Jack Johnson* (1844) and *The Struggles and Adventures of Christopher Tadpole at Home and Abroad* (1848). There is a memoir by Edmund Yates in the 1860 edition of Smith's *Mont Blanc* (first published, as *The Story of Mont Blanc*, 1853).

53. John Thurtell (1794–1824), notorious gambler and swindler, murdered a solicitor named William Weare in 1823. Thurtell was hanged, and remained a sort of popular hero for some time.

54. Bayard Taylor (1825–78), an American, wrote travel books, novels, and poems, and translated *Faust* in the original metres (1870–71). There is a biography by Albert H. Smyth (1896).

LIST OF WORKS QUOTED
BY ACTON IN *PROSTITUTION*

COOPER, *Sir* ASTLEY. Lectures on the principles and practice of surgery, as delivered in the theatre of St Thomas's hospital. Second edition. *London, F. C. Westley,* 1830.

Eleventh report of the Medical Officer of the Privy Council: with appendix: 1868. *London, H.M.S.O.* 1869. *Reports from Commissioners,* 1868–9, XXXII. 4217.

ESQUIROS, ALPHONSE. Les Vierges folles. [Third edition.] *Paris, Delavigné,* 1842.

HILL, MATTHEW DAVENPORT. Suggestions for the repression of crime, contained in charges delivered to grand juries of Birmingham. *London, John W. Parker,* 1857.

JEANNEL, J. De la prostitution dans les grandes villes au dix-neuvième siècle et de l'extinction des maladies vénériennes. *Paris, Baillière,* 1868.

PARENT-DUCHÂTELET, A.-J.-B. De la prostitution dans la ville de Paris, considérée sous le rapport de l'hygiène publique, de la morale et de l'administration. Troisième édition, complétée . . . par . . . A. Trebuchet [et] Poirat-Duval. *Paris, Baillière,* 1857. 2 tom.

Report from the Select Committee of the House of Lords on the Contagious Diseases Act, 1866; together with the proceedings of the committee, minutes of evidence, and appendix. 1868. *Sessional Papers,* 1867–8, XXX. 136.

Report from the Select Committee on Contagious Diseases Act (1866); together with the proceedings of the committee, minutes of evidence, and appendix. 1869. *Reports from Committees,* 1868–9, II. 306.

TAYLOR, BAYARD. Northern travel: summer and winter pictures of Sweden, Lapland, and Norway. *London, Sampson Low,* 1858.

TENNYSON, ALFRED. Idylls of the King. *London, Edward Moxon & Co.,* 1859.

Note: Pope's lines quoted by Acton on p. 115 are most conveniently to be found in the Twickenham edition of *The Poems of Alexander Pope,* ed. John Butt and others (1st edn, 1939 etc.; 2nd edn, 1953 etc.; 3rd edn, 1962 etc.), III. ii. 64 (and cf. VI. 377).

CHECK-LIST OF ACTON'S WORKS

I. BOOKS

A complete practical treatise on venereal diseases, and their immediate and remote consequences: including observations on certain affections of the uterus, attended with discharges. *London, Henry Renshaw,* 1841. pp. xxxii 410. 8vo.

A complete practical treatise on venereal diseases, *etc.* Atlas. *London, Henry Renshaw,* 1841. pp. [18]. pl. 8. oblong fol.

> Reviews: *Lancet,* 1840–41, II. 342–5; *London Medical Gazette,* n.s. II (1840–41), 475–7; *Medico-Chirurgical Review,* XXXV (1841), 26–31.

[Another edition.] A complete practical treatise on venereal diseases, *etc.* First American edition, with additional illustrations, *etc. New York, J. S. Redfield,* 1846. pp. 334. pl. 8. 8vo.

[Another edition.] *New York, J. S. Redfield,* 1848. pp. 333. pl. 7. 8vo.

[Another edition.] A practical treatise on diseases of the urinary and generative organs (in both sexes). Second edition. *London, John Churchill,* 1851. pp. [i] viii [i] 693. 8vo.

> Reviews: *British and Foreign Medico-Chirurgical Review,* VIII (1851), 182–203; *Lancet,* 1851, I. 436; *London Journal of Medicine,* III (1851), 644–53, 709–17; *London Medical Gazette,* n.s. XII (1851), 1039–43.

[Another edition.] *New York, J. S. Redfield,* 1852. pp. 459. pl. 7. 8vo.

[Another edition.] Third edition. *London, John Churchill,* 1860. pp. xxxii 608. pl. 11. 8vo.

> Reviews: *British Medical Journal,* 1860, 960–1; *Lancet,* 1861, I. 413–15, 463–7; *Medical Times and Gazette,* 1860, II. 617.

Prostitution in relation to public health; forming the introductory chapter to the second edition of the treatise on syphilis. Reprinted for private circulation. *London, J. Churchill,* 1851. pp. 24. 8vo.

> Review: *Medical Times,* XXIII (1851), 297–8.

[A translation.] De la prostitution considerée au point de vue de l'hygiène publique. Traduit de l'anglais par Alph. Guérard. *Annales d'hygiène publique et de médecine légale,* XLVI (1851), 39–71.

The functions and disorders of the reproductive organs in youth, in

PROSTITUTION

adult age, and in advanced life: considered in their physiological, social, and psychological relations. *London, John Churchill*, 1857. pp. vi [i] 108. 8vo.

Reviews: *British and Foreign Medico-Chirurgical Review*, XX (1857), 176–7; *British Medical Journal*, 1857, 279–80; *Lancet*, 1857, I. 556–7; *Medical Times and Gazette*, XXXV (1857), 492–3.

[Another edition.] Second edition. *London, John Churchill*, 1858. pp. viii [i] 123. 8vo.

[Another edition.] The functions and disorders of the reproductive organs in childhood, youth, adult age, and advanced life considered in their physiological, social, and moral relations. Third edition. *London, John Churchill*, 1862. pp. xvii 218. 8vo.

Reviews: *British and Foreign Medico-Chirurgical Review*, XXX (1862), 164–5; *Lancet*, 1862, I. 518–19; *Medical Times and Gazette*, 1862, I. 488.

[A translation.] Fonctions et désordres des organes de la génération chez l'enfant, le jeune homme, l'adulte et le viéllard sous le rapport physiologique, social et moral. Traduit de l'anglais sur la 3. éd. *Paris, V. Masson*, 1863. pp. iii 366. 8vo.

Review: *La Gazette médicale de Paris*, XVIII (1863), 476–8.

[Another edition.] The functions and disorders of the reproductive organs, *etc.* Fourth edition. *London, John Churchill*, 1865. pp. xiv 243. 8vo.

[Another edition.] *Philadelphia, Lindsay & Blakiston*, 1865. pp. 254. 8vo.

[Another edition.] Second American edition. *Philadelphia, Lindsay & Blakiston*, 1867. pp. xiv 291. 8vo.

[Another edition.] Fifth edition. *London, J. & A. Churchill*, 1871. pp. xvi 262. 8vo.

[Another edition.] Sixth edition. *London, J. & A. Churchill*, 1875. pp. xii 266. 8vo.

[Another edition.] Sixth edition. *Philadelphia, P. Blakiston*, 1883. pp. xii 267. 8vo.

[Another edition.] *Philadelphia, P. Blakiston*, 1888. pp. xii 263. 8vo.

[Another edition.] *Philadelphia, P. Blakiston*, 1894. pp. xii 263. 8vo.

Prostitution, considered in its moral, social, & sanitary aspects, in London and other large cities: with proposals for the mitigation and prevention of its attendant evils. *London, John Churchill*, 1857. pp. ix [i] 189. 8vo.

Reviews: *British and Foreign Medico-Chirurgical Review*, XXI

(1858), 388–415; *Medical Times and Gazette*, XXXVI (1857), 458; *Sanitary Review and Journal of Public Health*, III (1857–58), 327–35.

[Another edition.] Prostitution, considered in its moral, social, and sanitary aspects, in London and other large cities and garrison towns: with proposals for the control and prevention of its attendant evils. Second edition. *London, John Churchill*, 1870. pp. xvi 302. 8vo.

Reviews: *British and Foreign Medico-Chirurgical Review*, XLVI (1870), 81–100; *Lancet*, 1870, I. 161–2.

The Contagious Diseases Act: shall the Contagious Diseases Act be applied to the civil population? Being a paper read before the Association of Medical Officers of Health, on Saturday, December 18th, 1869. *London, John Churchill*, 1870. pp. 36. 8vo.

II. CONTRIBUTIONS TO PERIODICALS, ETC.

On the advantages to be derived from the study of inoculation, in the investigation and treatment of the venereal disease. *Lancet*, 1839–40, I. 351–4.

Advantages of inoculation in the venereal disease. *Lancet*, 1839–40, I. 533–5.

A practical essay on the employment of mercury in syphilis. *Lancet*, 1839–40, I. 871–6.

Westminster Medical Society, Saturday, November 13, 1841. 'Mr Acton exhibited a new syringe. . . .' *Lancet*, 1841–42, I. 272–3. [Abstract]

Westminster Medical Society. . . . Case of secondary symptoms, principally consisting of condylomata, in a child eight years of age. *Lancet*, 1844, I. 201–2. [Abstract]

Observations on Dr Campbell's paper on congenite syphilis, in the first number of this journal. *Northern Journal of Medicine*, I (1844), 115–18. [Note by the editors, 118–19]

Aggravated case of eczema rubrum on the genital organs, mistaken for syphilis. *Lancet*, 1845, I. 10–11.

Constitutional syphilis in the father, a cause of repeated abortions, and subsequent infection of the fœtus, born at the full period, the mother remaining wholly free from disease; with observations. *London Medical Gazette*, n.s. I (1845), 164–6. [Abstract, discussion, and reply; also in *Lancet*, 1845, I. 651]

An account of a case of partial double monstrosity (Ischiopage Symelien

243

of Geoffroy Saint-Hilaire, Heteradelphia of Vrolik). *Medico-Chirurgical Transactions*, XXIX (1846), 103–6, 106*. pl. 1. [Also in *Lancet*, 1846, I. 337]

On the best means of disguising the taste of nauseous medicines. *Pharmaceutical Journal and Transactions*, V (1845–46), 502–5. [Also in *Lancet*, 1846, I. 603–4]

Can a nurse become affected with syphilis from suckling a child labouring under secondary symptoms? Instance bearing on the question. *Lancet*, 1846, II. 127–8.

On the causes, consequences, and treatment of indurated chancre. *Lancet*, 1846, II. 101–3, 609–10; 1847, I. 11–12, 220–2.

Contributions to the pathology, diagnosis, and treatment of venereal diseases. *Lancet*, 1846, I. 10–12, 69–70, 119–21, 179–80, 238–40, 326–8, 457–8, 627–9.

Observations on venereal diseases in the United Kingdom: from statistical reports in the army, navy, and merchant service, with remarks on the mortality from syphilis in the Metropolis; compiled from the official returns of the Registrar-General. *Lancet*, 1846, II. 369–72.

Diseases resembling the lues venerea and syphilis: an attempt at elucidating the complaints so called by John Hunter and Abernethy; with remarks on the diagnosis of such cases as occur at the present time. *Lancet*, 1847, II. 253–5.

Observations on a case supposed to prove that secondary symptoms are contagious and capable of transmission. *Lancet*, 1847, I. 508–10.

On the advantages of solutions of caoutchouc and gutta percha in protecting the skin against the contagion of animal poisons. *Lancet*, 1848, II. 598. [Also in *London Journal of Medicine*, I (1849), 108]

On the present condition and treatment of venereal diseases in Paris, from notes taken during a recent visit to the French metropolis. *Lancet*, 1850, II. 51–3.

Remarks on the present treatment of venereal diseases in the hospitals of Paris, as observed during a recent visit to that city. *London Medical Journal*, II (1850), 605–7. [Abstract, discussion, and reply]

[On the use of the speculum. Remarks at a meeting of the Royal Medical and Chirurgical Society.] *Lancet*, 1850, I. 702.

[On venereal ulcers. Remarks at a meeting of the Westminster Medical Society.] *London Journal of Medicine*, II (1850), 206–7.

Mr Acton on Mr Syme's operation for stricture. *London Medical Gazette*, XIII (1851), 86.

A sketch of the present condition and treatment of diseases of the urinary and generative organs in Paris. *Lancet*, 1854, I. 658–9; II. 7–8, 310–11.

On the modern treatment of diseases of the urinary and generative organs in Paris as compared with London, from notes lately taken in the French hospitals. *Lancet*, 1855, II. 543–5, 599–600; 1856, I. 36–8, 91–3.

Prostitution. *Transactions of the National Association for the Promotion of Social Science, 1857* (1858), 605–8. [Abstract]

Prostitution and visionary philanthropists. *Medical Times and Gazette*, XXXVII (1858), 279–80.

Public prostitution. *British Medical Journal*, 1858, 95–6.

Manufactured pasteboard splints. *Lancet*, 1859, II. 621.

Observations on illegitimacy in the London parishes of St Marylebone, St Pancras, and St George's, Southwark, during the year 1857; deduced from the returns of the Registrar-General. *Journal of the Statistical Society*, XXII (1859), 491–505.

Unmarried wet-nurses. *Lancet*, 1859, I. 175–6.

The death-drains at Brighton. *Lancet*, 1860, II. 522.

The drains of Brighton. *Lancet*, 1860, II. 570–1.

On the rarity and mildness of syphilis among the Belgian troops quartered in Brussels, as compared with its prevalence and severity among the foot guards in London. *Lancet*, 1860, I. 196–8. [Also in: *British Medical Journal*, 1860, 151–2; *Medical Times and Gazette*, 1860, I. 199–202; *Proceedings of the Royal Medical and Chirurgical Society*, III (1860), 175–80]

Child-murder and wet-nursing. *British Medical Journal*, 1861, I. 183–4.

Post-mortem examination of the late Lord Campbell. *Lancet*, 1861, I. 193–4.

Can syphilis be communicated by vaccination? *British Medical Journal*, 1862, I. 214–15. [Editorial comment, 207]

Personal experiences of an habitual traveller. *Lancet*, 1862, I. 210–11.

Small-pox among sheep. *Lancet*, 1862, II. 292–3.

Assumption of professional names to designate quack medicines. *Lancet*, 1863, I. 527.

Observations on venereal diseases, with suggestions for the amelioration of this army pestilence. *Royal Commission on the Sanitary State of the Army in India* (1863), I. 489–91.

[Evidence of Mr William Acton, M.R.C.S.] *Report from the Select Committee of the House of Lords on the Contagious Diseases Act, 1866* (1868), pp. 102–16.

Nitrate of silver injections in spermatorrhoea. *British Medical Journal*, 1868, II. 673.

Social dialectics. *British Medical Journal*, 1868, II. 153.

Is it inconsistent with the dignity of the profession to perform the duties which would be entailed on surgeons by the extension of the Contagious Diseases Act to the civil population? *Medical Times and Gazette*, 1870, I. 186–7.

Is it not incumbent on the medical profession to remove certain popular prejudices in reference to the Contagious Diseases Act? *British Medical Journal*, 1870, I. 350–1.

Shall we find that by the control of prostitution we have irretrievably lost in morality and gained not at all in health? *British Medical Journal*, 1870, II. 76–7.

Supposing the legislature should determine to recommend the introduction of the Contagious Diseases Act among the civil population, would it be possible and feasible to carry out its enactments in the metropolis? *Medical Times and Gazette*, 1870, I. 77. [Abstract. Discussion and reply, 77–8, 132–5]

The modern treatment of the advanced stages of constitutional syphilis. *British Medical Journal*, 1872, II. 186–7.

Whether the Contagious Diseases Acts shall be repealed, continued, or extended to the general population. *Medical Times and Gazette*, 1872, I. 207. [Abstract, discussion, and reply]

Is it politic to withhold the soldier's pay when in hospital? *Lancet*, 1873, I. 359–60.

Reflections on the possible motives for the Coram-street murder. *Lancet*, 1873, I. 115.

French testimony to the beneficial working of the Contagious Diseases Acts in England. *Lancet*, 1874, I. 107–8.

On the modern treatment of the advanced stages of constitutional syphilis. *British Medical Journal*, 1875, II. 258. [Abstract]

On the prevalence and severity of syphilis among troops quartered in London, as compared with the rarity of the disease among soldiers in the garrisons of Paris and Brussels; from observations, the result of a personal investigation made during the autumn of 1874. *Lancet*, 1875, I. 570–3. [Abstract. Also in: *British Medical Journal*, 1875, I. 522–4; *Medical Times and Gazette*, 1875, I. 507–13; *Proceedings of the Royal Medical & Chirurgical Society of London*, VII (1871–75), 345–50]

INDEX

ABRAHAM, James Johnston, 9 n.

accommodation houses, 26, 45–7, 105–6, 155, 165–7; number of, in London, 33, 38, 46

Acton, Edward, 8

Acton, Eizabeth, 8

Acton, William John: and Contagious Diseases Acts, 7, 8, and *pass.*; as campaigner, 7, 8, 16, 17, 22; as inventor, 11; birth, 8; career, 8 ff.; *Complete Practical Treatise on Venereal Diseases* (1841), 10, 241; death, 16; early life, 8–9; *Functions and Disorders of the Reproductive Organs* (1857), 11, 11–12, 241–2; list of his works, 241–6; medical training, 8–9; on Brighton's drainage, 15–16; on 'fallen women', 13, 25; on female sexuality, 12; on frequency of coitus, 12; on masturbation, 12; on quack advertisements, 9; on travelling, 14; *Prostitution* (1857), 7, 10, 11, 13, 13 n., 17, 18, 225–31, 242–3; reception of his work, 13–14, 225–31; reputation, 13–14, 16

Aldershot, 35, 56–8, 127, 128, 142, 153, 234

Aldershot Lock Hospital, 94–6, 127

Alhambra music-hall, 55, 236

Argyll Rooms, 50 f., 75, 170, 221–3, 235

army, 18, 21, 35, 56–8, 78, 79, 88–90, 92, 109, 110–11, 125, 151

Association for Promoting the Extension of the Contagious Diseases Act, 1866, to the Civil Population of the United Kingdom, 180, 239

Association for the Protection of Women, 129

BABY-FARMING, 25, 203–4

Barr, John Coleman, 35, 56, 127, 234

Bell, Benjamin, 9 n.

Belgium, 18, 245, 246

Berenger, Charles Random de, 234

Berlin, 18, 30, 37, 111, 224, 229–30

Bickersteth, Edward Henry, 191, 239

Bignell, Robert, 235

Blackwall parties, 62, 236

Board of Health, 15

Booth, Charles, 8 n.

Bracebridge, Samuel, 17, 18

Brewer, William, 30, 233

Brighton, 14, 15–16

British Medical Journal, 7, 14, 241–6 pass.

Brock, William, 191–2, 239

Brompton, 58, 62, 223

brothels, 33 ff., 53–4, 100 ff., 111, 149, 150, 152, 155, 164, 166, 182, 226; number of, in London, 33–4, 38

Busk, George, 79, 236

Butler, Josephine Elizabeth, 232

CAMBRIDGE, 55, 155

Campbell, John, first baron Campbell, 149

Charity Commissioners, 25

Cleugh, James, 9 n.

Colquhoun, Patrick, 17 n., 32, 233–4

247